Chapter 1

Life through a child's eyes
"Joy comes from the little victories, and is preferable to the fun that comes with ease and the pursuit of pleasure."
(Lawana Blackwell)

We begin when I am 8 years old, the firstborn of two Scottish professional immigrant parents, growing up in a suburb in eastern Sydney. My world was wonderful. My life was carefree, untroubled and perfect, free from any distress, apprehension or disappointment. Being a parent now, I can see that children don't see life realistically, they see only its innocence and potential, they see it completely through eyes coloured by their limited experiences and knowledge. As adults, we forget how great this is. We are moulded by circumstances, hurts and fears.

At 8 years old I saw my whole world as a true gift of discovery. My life was like a box of wrapped chocolates, an offering that I had the opportunity to unpack and explore, piece by piece. From the security of my familiar world, I wanted only to investigate every aspect of it. I had an inquisitive nature, and was eager to learn and explore. I would not let anything pass me by.

In the early '70s, the world was vastly different to the one we live in today. We were living in a new country. Men had landed on the moon for the first time. Television was not corrupted by evil and horrid visions of disaster and doom, like 9/11. They were exciting times.

I could buy big, bronzed, crispy potato scallops made from thin slabs of potatoes for 2 cents each, and I loved them! It was a time, where adventurous and energetic kids, like me, preferred to roam the streets and play outside in the sun. I despised the rainy days, they trapped me like a prisoner - in my own home.

My friends and I would terrorize the neighbourhoods with our re-enactments of fantasy cowboy and Indian battles. Each of us would run and hide behind large trees, and roll in thickly flowered garden beds to gain the best vantage points for our territorial wars. We fired our Winchester long-barrelled rifles, loaded our large wooden bows, ready to shoot the imaginary long-feathered arrows.

At times, we actually had what we considered the real deal; we wore heavily intricately patterned steel toy guns, which dangled from leather gun holsters slung low on our narrow hips. We also spent hours building four-wheeled go carts, using broken discarded pram wheels and old pieces of discarded wood that were strewn next to the roadside. These makeshift carts were held together with whatever we could find - usually off-cuts of discarded string.

Treacherous and risky by today's standards, but, it was so much fun. Not even the painful bouts of gravel rash or having to scrub my legs and arms with a steel brush to remove the gravel after I crashed could deter me from perilously pitching my body uncontrollably down the steep hills. I also played in the surrounding heavily wooded parks; I rolled in the grass, climbed the magnificent old trees and splashed through the swirling pools of water. In the early years of my life, there were no computers, Play Stations or iPods. We had to make our own fun.

I never imagined that the only life I knew could be shattered so easily. I was completely unaware of the fragility of life or the profound effect just one event could make on a person psychologically, emotionally and physically. Or how one event could radically change the course of a life - my life. Or, how it could transform my beliefs and dreams, and turn them into something unspeakable.

I was about to enter into a vile, horrifying nightmare which would shatter everything real in my life. It would destroy my familiar sanctuary, devastate my wellbeing and change me forever.

It was a high counsel that I once heard given to a young person, "Always do what you are afraid to do."

Ralph Waldo Emerson

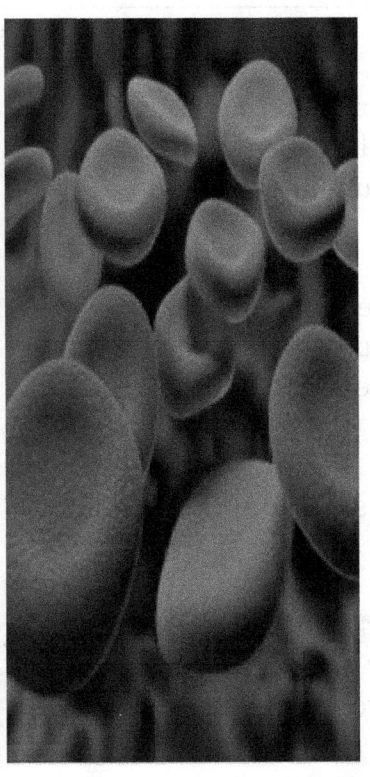

Hepatitis C (HCV) is what is known as a Blood-borne virus that affects the liver. It is transmitted via blood to blood contact, through sharing injecting equipment, unsterile piercing and tattooing. Although household transmission is rare, it is possible if you share toothbrushes, razors or tweezers. Sexual transmission is also uncommon but can occur if there is blood to blood contact.

If you require any further information contact the Hepatitis Council in your state.

Or visit my website
www.hepcandme.com.au

From Torment to Freedom, Copyright 2012 by Laurie Smyth. All rights to this story and to this work and this book in all mediums, are reserved by Laurie Smyth, the author and writer of this work. This book is sold on the condition that no part of this material can be replicated, reproduced or transmitted in any form electronically, mechanically, photocopying, recording or any other form of social medium without the permission of Laurie Smyth. This work is protected in accordance with the Copyright Act 1968 and all applicable amendments and international agreements. Permission request can be sent to **lasmyth@hotmail.com** Or visit www.hepcandme.com.au

First edition 2012-1-30
ISBN   **978-0-9871866-0-7**
Front and Back cover designed by Ray Smyth
Thanks to Adam Duncan for reviewing the book content

Acknowledgments

To the many people, who helped and supported me through this long journey. Your input into my life has been uplifting and inspiring. I am more grateful than you will ever know, thank you.

Betty, my dear friend, I wouldn't be the person I am today if our paths had not crossed. Thank you, you helped save me from the darkness that loomed and threatened to overwhelm me.

For those who stood courageously by my side, supporting and praying for me I am eternally grateful.

To my family, who have travelled this life with me, I love you, now and always. I am indebted to you for your loyal support and encouragement. You are the pillars around my life that constantly sustain me.

I dedicate this book to two men who have fought valiantly beside me, who meticulously picked up the pieces of my brokenness and repeatedly made me whole again. Men who enthusiastically and wholehearted supported the writing of this story, cheering me on from the sidelines and encouraging me when I lost my momentum.

This book is for you

        Thank you and I love you both.
        To my father and my husband.

From Torment to freedom

It is the fire of suffering that brings forth the gold of Godliness.
Madame Guyon

It is not the critic who counts, nor the man who points out how the strong man stumbled, or where the doer of deeds could have done them better. The credit belongs to the man who is actually in the arena, whose face is marred by dust and sweat and blood; who strives valiantly; who errs and comes short again and again; who knows great enthusiasms, great devotions; who spends himself in a worthy cause; who, at the best, knows in the end the triumph of high achievement, and who, at the worst, if he fails, at least fails while daring greatly, so that his place shall never be with those timid souls who know neither victory nor defeat.

Theodore Roosevelt

Authors note.

This book is a personal expedition, a very individual voyage. It is a true portrayal and illustration of my life and the choices I made. I, like you, am simply a lone solitary ship trying to navigate through the tumultuous and sometimes peaceful oceans of life. My journey of 48 years has now provided me with a distinct and very personal purpose - the creation of this book and the message I hope it brings. I welcome you to my unique insight into a world fraught with inarguable hardship. It describes my personal war. A war I waged upon an insidious enemy and the defences I used to try and overcome my adversary. It also demonstrates a life, which encompasses unbelievable expectation, faith, as well as, revealing the subtle elegance and beauty that life holds.

Life has tested me on so many levels; it has presented complex challenges, gruelling problems, senseless tragedies and unanswered prayers. Not unlike your own journey, I imagine. Yet, if my choices were different, I would not be the person I am today.

I anticipate this story may take you on your own personal journey, a journey of personal awakening and self-discovery. I hope my story

provides you with some alternative strategies and inspiration. I have found that the most unusual and unexpected paths offered in life can lead to many mystifying, yet life-changing, outcomes.
This book exposes the trials, the hurts and the fears that I lived through. I am who I am, because of what life has thrown at me. Life is tough on so many levels.

I entered this world, like you, with an undefined life. I later defined it by my choices. It is sometimes a circus, a minefield, a marathon and a dance. It can be whatever we choose it to be. If I could impart some wisdom to you, it would be to live your life with authentic passion and purpose. All your worldly tributes and accolades are easily forgotten, the real legacy you leave behind is the creation of genuine relationships. Create lasting relationships built on mutual respect, acceptance, trust and love; these are the true relationships that last the test of time. These relationships will be what carry you through the hard times of your life.

Would I like to change any aspect of my life? Yes, of course I would, but, none of us have the chance to go backwards. I hope as you move through the years of your life, you can really see the world for all its offerings, its beauty and capabilities, not just the suffering and difficulties you have faced.

I hope that this book can bring a message of hope and peace to you. Settle back in your favourite chair, grab a nice cup of steamy hot chocolate, and enjoy the journey I am about to take you on.
So lets begin....

Chapter 2

Destiny, can it be changed?
I know God will not give me anything I can't handle. I just wish that He didn't trust me so much.
~Mother Teresa

In 1971, when I was 8 years old, my world was struck by a large meteorite. An event so devastating that it would leave huge craters and turbulent storms in my life for a long time to come.
School was over for the day and I started the slow trek home. The winter's afternoon sun touched my skin with its warm yellow rays of light; its soft smooth fingers caressed my face, it revitalized my spirits after my tedious day at school. To me, school was a laborious task. I found it unstimulating and uninteresting. I preferred to amuse myself with more recreational activities, such as the development of daring acts on the steel monkey bars, rather than cultivating the concepts of Math's or English and the gaining of wisdom.

My route home funnelled me past a local small corner store and, my favourite, the local fish-and-chip shop. It was the finest place I had stumbled upon in all my years. The owner, a middle aged friendly Italian man, served me my order of 5 well-done, crispy, golden brown, yummy potato scallops. I was a creature of habit, routinely visiting this haunt on my way home. I loved to smother these treats in a lather of salt and vinegar. Then, I would slowly devour them, savouring every mouthful as I continued to walk home through my favourite playground, the local park.

This park was only 200 meters from my home, and bordered the road that led directly to my street and the football field, which I also played on. My mother didn't like me to play or walk through this place. She regularly argued with me over my choice to continue to hang out there, but, it was the shortest and simplest route home. Plus, it was the coolest place to play.

I rounded the corner, and the front door of my house came into view. I quickly rubbed my face on my navy blue school jumper and wiped my hands on my skirt to remove and evidence of my feast.

As I drew near to my house, I could hear my new young brother screaming; his shrill voice spoiled my buoyant frame of mind. I was sure that he knew exactly when I was near and timed his ear-piercing cries just for my approach. I drew a deep breath, sighed, and stealthily entered the house. My aim was to quietly creep past him and reach the tranquillity of my room unnoticed.

My frazzled mother, temporarily house-bound from her professional career, sat directly in my path. She tried everything to soothe and calm him, but he would not stop screaming. I empathised with her. I understood the strain she felt, as the constant noise wore me down, and I wasn't with him 24 hours a day like she was. He was a difficult child, who limited her ability to complete even the most menial of tasks. There was no way I could slip past her unnoticed. As I entered the room, her eyes met mine. Unspoken, yet unmistakable words passed between us "help me, can you give me a break PLEASE". I dropped my bag on the floor and offered to assist her, reaching out to take my tiny brother from her arms.

She quickly moved to the kitchen, to get her purse and asked if I would go to the shop for her. She needed potatoes for dinner and had no other way of getting them. I jumped at the opportunity, happy to once again be away from the household commotion and the constant bombardment of sounds. I gathered her small string bag from the kitchen counter, placed the coins she handed me in my pocket, and walked happily out the door. Behind me, I heard her apprehensive, rapidly fading voice, her instructions clear and precise: "do not go through the park". Over my shoulder, I yelled back "I won't" and cheerfully skipped off down the road. Relieved to be released from the constant volley which my home life now offered, I cheerfully walked to my destination with her coins jingling in my pocket.

As I stood at the counter to purchase my chosen potatoes, I longingly eyed the large heavily-laden lolly jars, directly positioned in my line of vision; they taunted me, called out to me. I wished I had some spare money for a couple of those deliciously chewy chocolate-covered cobbers, but, it was not to be. I turned and left the store, without any chocolate. Instead, five potatoes sat snugly in the coloured string bag as I carried them thoughtlessly homeward. For the second time today, I found myself sauntering through the heavily wooded gardens of the park. This time I carried an essential part of the evening meal instead of my usual school pack. I playfully swung the potato laden string bag back and forth and enjoyed the luxuriant fragrance of the flowers that surrounded me.

Long shadows moved in menacing patterns and darkened my familiar garden, as the clouds played hide and seek with the sun. The large, leafy branches from the weeping willows spilled over onto the footpath like a cascading waterfall. As I sauntered down the path, I could hear the leaves of these majestic trees as they rustled in the gentle breeze. In front of me lay the big exposed concrete water pipes my friends and I regularly played in. We would carelessly splash in the ankle deep cold water, as it gently flowed into the pipes.

A vision flickered; my mind displayed the last stored memory of this exact location. Pictures of my friends and I, as we joyfully played, talked and laughed. We searched out and ensnared tiny tadpoles with the hope of fostering a pet frog. Unfortunately, I was not a great nurturer; I was more in the funeral director category, as mine always died a day after capture, requiring a burial ceremony.

In the distance, my friend's house emerged, my task now nearly complete, and I would return to my home and all its commotion. The last of the big overhanging trees bordering the creek loomed in front of me. My mind returned to the scene of my mother and brother waiting at home. If I was lucky, my friend might see me, which would delay my homecoming; this thought brought a smile to my lips, and memories of our ventures flashed through my mind.

My mother's words revisited me, haunting me. Her clear instruction not to go through the park awakened a new pang of guilt within me. Here I was doing exactly what I was told not to do. I just could not understand why she didn't like this park; she discouraged me from playing here more often than not. But I just loved being in its presence. The wonders and secrets it held, its beauty, the flowers, the trees, the water, all of it held such delight and charm for me.

My vivid imagination frequently engulfed my whole attention and this instance was no different. I imagined walking in an open field, the sun light illuminated the path before me, it swept over my face and warmed my skin with its beams. A gentle wind brushed and toyed with my long black hair, it blew lingering strands around my face. A shiny black horse gently nudged my hand, as he sought affection. For me, there could be nothing better than getting lost in my fantasy world.

Unexpectedly, I was wrenched from my invented safe playground, momentarily startled, by a young man in his early 20's, as he sprung from behind a large weeping willow. He stood directly in front of me, deliberately blocking my path. What did he want? He looked scary. Behind him was the safety of the road and I could see the steady stream of traffic as commuters returned home after a day at work. The details of my friend's safe haven, right in front of me within reach, but, my destiny was about to change right there, right then.

Your thoughts are the architects of your destiny.

David O. McKay

Chapter 3

Overwhelming fear

"When a resolute young fellow steps up to the great bully, the world, and takes him boldly by the beard, he is often surprised to find it comes off in his hand, and that it was only tied on to scare away the timid adventurers".
Ralph Waldo Emerson

In that split second, I realised I was in serious trouble. The man's dishevelled appearance and his expression alerted me to pending danger. My inexperienced mind was unable to process the details of the imminent threat, or identify the situation, or access any potential possibilities. But, I felt real fear for the first time in my life, not like when I was on the rides at the show; this was deep, earth-shattering fear.

Uncontrollable tremors advanced from my feet and swept over my whole body. Water welled in my eyes and cascaded down my cheeks. He stepped closer to me, his eyes wild and alert. He raised his hand and thrust a large, shiny knife in front of my face. The blade was long and jagged on one side, but it was the length of the blade and the sharp, pointed tip that really frightened me.

My mother's warning echoed in the recesses of my mind. Why had I not heeded her voice? Was I going to die? Was he going to kill me? Maybe stab me with that threatening knife? Why else would he grab me? Somewhere, deep within me, a tiny voice rose up. Sounds tumbled from my lips. My alert ears heard the softly spoken words. A question, I wondered where it came from, then I realised it was me speaking, as the words echoed in my ears, "please don't hurt me, my mother is waiting for me, and she needs these potatoes for dinner".

He looked deep into my eyes as he assessed me. Our eyes met and held for a long thoughtful moment. My mind completely blank, yet my body fully alert, as it waited for any response. He roughly reached forward and grabbed my arm, indenting and marking the skin just below my shoulder. My arm protested, under the pressure of his fingers, as they dug deeply into my flesh. He viciously forced my body to turn 180 degrees, to face the way I had just travelled.

This movement jerked my head, and I found myself momentarily disorientated, temporarily stunned, as pain shot through my jaw and my teeth snapped sharply together. My vision blurred and my legs became slightly unsteady, causing me to stumble. He heaved me upwards and pulled me close to his side, my body momentarily touched his lightly clad mass.

My heart galloped like a wild horse in my chest, as irrepressible and uncontrollable sobs escaped from deep within me. My body's natural impulses were forced into submission by his harsh coarse statements, telling me to shut up, and, keep moving, or something really bad was going to happen. My eight year old body succumbed to his oversized hands, as he violently pulled me and forced me to go in an unwanted direction. My unstable, quivering legs moved forward on their own accord, as they carried me further from the safety I could see in the distance, as I looked longingly over my shoulder.

My limbs, half the size of his, couldn't move to accommodate his desired pace. His fingers dug deeply into my arm. I sharply cried out as a hot, searing pain shot like a bullet up into my shoulder. I searched his face, but could only see a relentless hunger, one I didn't understand.

He stepped towards me, his mouth close to my ear, his breathing laboured and his hot breath noticeably heavy with the smell of alcohol. He whispered, "move faster, or, I will hurt you right here." These words and the cold steel blade that he had placed on my tear-stained cheek forced me to move quicker. My mind reeled as it tried to compartmentalize what was happening. All my past experience and knowledge had taught me to respect my elders, simply because they knew better than children, but this just felt wrong.

These days, children are taught to be careful. Back then, there was no such thing as 'stranger danger', or campaigns about child safety, it wasn't really an issue in the '70s. What I did know was that this situation was wrong. He felt wrong. Everything in me wanted to run, but I couldn't. I was trapped like a tethered horse.

Maliciously, he tugged my arm, and again pain encouraged me to move faster. My arm throbbed from his constant pressure. Pain ricocheted from my shoulder all the way down to my clenched fist. I tried to internally rationalise where we were going. It appeared we were moving towards the back of the park, where a large wire fence separated the park from a local cemetery. Voiceless questions sat silently upon my lips. Where were we actually going? Why? What was he going to do to me? I dared not ask him, not wanting to anger him further. The knife was too big and far too threatening. I was in serious danger, and I didn't know what to do. I just wanted to see my family again. All of their faces gently hovered in front of my eyes, and were washed away with the tears that continued to silently fall.

My hand clung tightly to the string bag full of potatoes. Their weight provided comfort and solace in this dark moment. I lifted them up and drew them close to my body, hugging them tightly. I reflected on my last hopeful, yet previously unappreciated, family scene, and welcomed the picture of my mother as she nursed my crying brother. This heartening sight produced another flurry of quiet tears.
Our pace finally slowed, and I found myself in a unfamiliar place.

Before me stood a landscape full of thick, dense trees with light rustling foliage underneath. A tall wire fence dissected the trees, separating two very different landscapes. Seconds passed before I realized where I had been taken. I stood at the border between my favourite park and the dark cemetery.

The sturdy wire fence towered over me, an impossible mountain to climb with my unsteady legs. As I looked down, I saw a portion of the wire fence folded back, lifted slightly. This would allow limited access to the cemetery beyond. I was physically dragged to this entry point, then flung to the ground, and forced onto my uncovered knees.

A rough, distant voice provided specific instructions as to how I was to go under the fence, and wait on the other side. I felt frozen in time, unable to move a muscle, anesthetized, but still wide awake; able to hear, feel and see everything. What was he going to do to me? Why here? Where was my protector? Why was no one here to help me?

There was no other choice. I had to keep moving. Slowly, I threw the bag of potatoes under the fence, then started to manoeuvre my body head first into the grounds of the cemetery. The leaves softened the ground for me as I dragged myself through the gap, using my hands and elbows like pulleys. Once I was nearly through, I felt the coldness of the steel blade as it was placed on the back of my leg. This prevented me from standing up or going any further, so, I lay face down in the dirt and waited, whilst my hands searched and found the comfort of the bag of potatoes.

He quickly joined me. As I stood up, it dawned on me; I now stood in the creepy, ominous cemetery. I recalled a familiar memory; a more positive and friendly occasion, when my friends and I rode our bikes on the concrete paths and manicured lawns as we explored the rows of headstones. However, the tales of macabre and horror that we shared quickly overrode the positive memories. These horror stories now taunted me. I always thought the place creepy and a bit eerie, especially the open and damaged grave sites. This place really scared me, and being here completely frightened me.

Fear and panic overrode every other emotion and thought I had; fear of being left here, to die a horrible unknown death, and panic of never being found or seeing my family again. I was pulled deeper into the ominous grave yard. Terror and dread grew more pronounced, with every step I took into this ancient burial ground. Out of the blue, his demeanour changed. Enthusiasm radiated from him, his tone mischievous, amused, his eyes intense, hungry and determined. This change in him confused me, it scared me.

Whatever was going to happen was going to happen now. I could feel it. I tried to back away from him, but I was too slow, he grabbed me and tossed me like a rag doll to the ground. The light foliage and hard clay ground dug into my back and scratched my legs as I landed. My skirt lifted and displayed my underwear, and my uncovered legs slightly splayed open. For a split second, I felt completely disorientated.

Adrenalin surged through my veins, enabling me to hastily try and get up. I knew I had to run, had to get as far away from this place as possible. I fought to bring my legs together and stand, but my 8 year old reactions were not skillful or practiced enough for the strength and experience of a 20 year old man. He was fast and determined.

He pushed me backwards, and grabbed both of my legs with his hands, and yanked them fully open. I shrieked in disagreement as I tried to scramble backwards away from him, but my movements were fruitless.

He overpowered me, and threw me on my back. His sizeable body, advantageously pinned me to the ground, beneath him, whilst he positioned himself purposefully between my legs, locking them in a compromising and open position. He victoriously smiled, as his eyes met mine. He knew he had won. I felt hopeless and overpowered. My peripheral vision enabled me to see that he had placed the knife within reach, near my face, but I was too scared to move, frozen, unable to think rationally.

His hand slowly reached between my legs. I felt his fingers as they explored my body, then abruptly he ripped off my underpants. I was completely exposed, vulnerable in every way. I just wanted my daddy. Where was he? Why couldn't he save me? He had protected me before, why not now? Why was this happening to me? What had I ever done to this man? Why did he want to hurt me like this?

He knelt between my legs and stared at me, thoughtfully reflecting on the picture he had created. Time stood still. I no longer looked at him. I closed my eyes tightly, not wanting to see anything anymore. What would be would be. If I died here now, I was ready. I knew that it would all be over then, no pain, no hurt, all of this done, finished.

I heard him as he unbuckled his jeans. I felt his body heat merge with mine as he came closer to his target. I heard a disgusting sound of spitting, and I felt the wetness as it struck me between the thighs. An unidentified scream rose from the depths of my being. It passed my lips as an immense, hot searing pain struck me, and I was unceremoniously and unsympathetically ripped open and left bleeding.

My physical attack was over in minutes, the mental pain would last a lot longer, and the scars would run very deep, not only for me, but for him also. He was done. It was over, but I was too shocked to move. Every muscle in my body ached. Light traces of blood pooled beneath me. I was suspended in time, caught between each second as the hammer steadily pounded the lower half of my body. I opened my eyes to see him towering over me, standing tall. His eyes pierced mine, searching intently for some thing unknown to me. I wasn't aware of it at the time, but I suppose he used this time to consider and review his options. He had a major decision to make. Endless and immeasurable seconds ticked by, our eyes locked in a silent struggle.

I noticed his shoulders slump slightly, the tension in his body released, as if a profound burden that had once weighed heavy upon him was decisively and completely removed. Hastily, he retreated from me and quickly dressed himself, unable to look at me any longer. Fully clothed, he leant towards me, grabbed my hand and pulled me to my feet. Offhandedly, he instructed me to tidy myself up. We silently walked side by side towards the hole in the fence.

My legs quivered beneath me, they screamed out in pain with every step. My stomach tossed, every muscle trembled. My whole focus was on the distant hole in the fence and what lay beyond it - my home and my family. I knew my freedom lay on the other side of the steel wall that held me captive, and every step I took brought me closer to my escape from this nightmare, from this evil vile man and what he had done.

I clearly saw the hole in the fence line and my pace quickened, as did my heart beat. I visualized my release. I could feel it, I could see it and I craved it. A sharp tug, and the searing pain it caused interrupted my focused escape. Again, I was forced to look at him. He glared at me with what appeared to me to be hatred. His dark eyes penetrated deep into my inner being. I felt tiny rivulets of water as they ran slowly down my cheeks, as fear threatened to overtake me again. He finally spoke. I heard a calm voice this time, and the words which told me to "go", and as a passing comment, he told me to not forget to tell my mother.

I searched his face, scanning for the truth. Was this a trick? I didn't have to think about it for too long, something in his face confirmed his words. I believed him, and I ran. I ran like a wind that swept through a corn field, flattening everything in its path. My bruised and battered legs cramped and screamed in pain, but still I did not stop. I was ecstatic. My shackles had been removed, broken, and my unencumbered feet moved swiftly, taking me away from that decaying place. I was on my way home, alive.

I felt euphoric when I reached my house. I didn't care that my brother was still screaming, I embraced the comfort that this familiarity brought. When I reached my frantically pacing mother, I was dirty, covered in dried mud and spots of blood, leaves bonded to my unruly messy hair. My dirt-covered face was smeared with deep tear stained rivulets, resembling roads on a map. She looked at me perceptively. I didn't have to speak; she somehow knew. I presented all the potatoes to her, for I had lost none. Anxious tears flowed from her eyes, as I allowed her warm safe arms to engulf and comfort me. She held me close for a long extended moment. I couldn't believe I was home, alive.

If you do not hope, you will not find what is beyond your hopes.

St. Clement of Alexandra

Chapter 4

An unbearable task

"As we are liberated from our own fear, our presence automatically liberates others."
Nelson Mandela

I was taken to the hospital and the formalities began. I was poked and prodded, then sent to the police station so I could formalise a statement. I wasn't sure if I had the strength to talk about it all over again. All I really wanted to do was curl up and go to sleep and forget the day ever happened.

A few hours after the assault, my mother and I were notified that the police had located a suspect, and we were again summoned to the police station, this time to identify the man who attacked me. My father had been called shortly after I returned home, but was stuck in the long traffic jams with thousands of other noisy, impatient Sydney commuters as they all tried to exit the city to return home. I wanted him there to support me, to hold my hand as I went back to the police station, but I didn't know whether his presence would have been a blessing or would have caused more of a crisis.

The never-ending event just seemed to go on and on, when really all I wanted to do was just curl up in the corner. I kept trying to put the incident away somewhere out of my mind, but as I constantly retold the story to strangers, as well as being shunted and forced to do things I didn't really want to do, the vivid pictures flooded through my mind.

I first spotted him as I walked escorted down a long narrow hallway. He quietly stood apart from the other casually dressed men, against a wall, in a small glass lined room. None of these other men held my focus, in fact I barely saw them. My eyes were instantly drawn to him, the man I knew to be my assailant. Fear welled up inside me and I drew close to my mother, seeking her protection.

I was met by a woman in a blue uniform who quickly ushered us into an adjacent, small, undecorated plain room, where I could no longer see him. Pangs of anxiety, terror and panic blazed through my body. Sweat glistened on my upper lip and exploded across my palms. My stomach stirred, like I had swallowed hundreds of fluttering butterflies. I didn't want to do this; I just wanted to go home.

The calm, unpretentious police officer assigned to be my escort dutifully informed me that I had to enter the unfurnished, formal room where five men stood, and pick out the man. Her words chilled me to the core, my mind and body in total harmony, one goal, to get me away from this God-forsaken place.

In the '70s, there was no one-way glass or sheltered hidden rooms for victims to stand in, to conceal them and protect them from the glares of the suspects in this kind of line up. The process was conducted all out in the open, the victim, me, had to walk amongst the suspects, confront each person individually, and point out the person.

Fear overwhelmed me. My legs trembled uncontrollably. Vibrations caused my whole body to shudder wildly. I thought I may collapse at any moment, and I struggled with this predicament. I knew I had to go in there, but my body and mind were unwilling to react to this fact. Words of encouragement were whispered gently in my ear.

Could I embrace them, step into that room, and do what was required of me? I searched for solace in my mother's face, but she was unable to assist me. I felt lost, abandoned, alone and scared. A hand gently rested on my shoulder and guided me out of my sanctuary, into the arena. A blue-clad gladiator stood by my side, offering protection, and directed my every move. The weight on my shoulder encouraged me, but did not ease the turmoil that raged within me.

I unsteadily stood in the centre of the room, unable to look at the men who stood before me. Fear and anxiety terrorized me; they struck me in waves, threatening to engulf me. The perceptive, discerning eyes of my guide held mine. They reached out from a distance and offered support. The rules of engagement were clearly explained. I knew my task; I was required to pick him out from the line up in front of me. Simple, whilst they were just words floating on the air. Putting them into practice would be a different story.

Laurie Smyth

I struggled hard not to look into the menacing faces of the men, but my eyes were drawn to them anyway. It didn't take long. I knew exactly where he stood. I smelt him, sensed him, his presence overpowered the room. My hand automatically lifted and a finger shot out. It rapidly fired the fatal blow. Relief washed over me. I turned to leave, as I knew it was over. But not quite.

My new guardian became a traitor, demanding that I actually touch the man, to ensure that I had chosen the right person. I was horrified, sickened and disgusted at this request. I didn't want to touch him or feel him on my skin. I stared at my one-time ally, dumbstruck. A strong, sharp, bitter taste flowed evenly into my mouth. It made me hyper-salivate and forced me to swallow rapidly. My stomach revisited my afternoon snack. The taste, a bitter tang - I would never enjoy those potato scallops again.

The quiet stillness of the room was shattered by my father's ear-piercing cries. Uniforms swarmed around him, preventing him from accessing me, his angry roars directed at my attacker. I feared, if my father was freed from his blue confinement, he may actually kill this man. I couldn't hold on any longer, the room swam ominously around me. I was like a fish confined to a small tank, and I wanted my freedom. I had done everything required of me so far. Why did I need to touch him? I wanted my dad to take me far away from this place, but he was trapped in a sea of bodies with no possibility of escape. My father's disturbance was only a temporarily interruption to the task. I was still required to touch the man. I anxiously wondered what would happen if he grabbed me again.

I suddenly felt fragmented, disoriented. I experienced an out-of-body sensation, the connection between my brain and my body vanished. My mind drifted carelessly into a cloud. I would wake up and this day would start over. But a gentle nudge in the small of my back brought me sharply back to the reality of where I was...... the line up of young men in front of me.

My legs moved robotically towards the man. Somewhere from within me, I felt the tip of my pointed finger touch the soft part of his belly. I was still too small to reach his chest or shoulder, as I would have preferred. My hand swiftly and unexpectedly recoiled. I hastily retreated to the safety of the officer. As soon as I stepped back, I was wordlessly steered from the room, and the rest of that night became a blur in my memory.

"Sometimes the littlest things in life are the hardest to take. You can sit on a mountain more comfortably than on a tack."

~Author Unknown

Chapter 5

Seasons begin to change

"I call heaven and earth to record this day against you, that I have set before you life and death, blessing and cursing:"
Deuteronomy 30:19

Hours flowed mindlessly into days, then weeks, then months. Life did not have the same flavour as it did before, my essence seriously tainted by an experience that would spoil my life's value forever. My previous, carefree, relaxed manner, now a behaviour of the past. I became nervous and anxious all the time, so I stayed at home and hardly ventured out. I played imaginary games in the back yard alone, burying myself in my deeply darkened, sometimes empty, thoughts.

The day that was supposed to change my life, with its promise of justice, arrived. People around me thought that this would be the end of the saga, and I would return to my previously happy and contented self. However, I was not a robot that could be switched on and off at will. The feelings I felt were like destructive forces that wanted to crush me. I tried, but I just couldn't understand or deal with any of it. The situation was far too extreme and complex for my 8 year old brain to cope with or sort out. I certainly knew the way I felt would not change just because the man was caught and we were in court, seeking a conviction.

It was my turn to give evidence. I sat nervously in the wooden witness box, next to a man wearing a suit and a funny looking wig. My clammy, moist fingers squeezed and pinched the skin on my forearm. My heart beat fast and loud as questions were fired at me like bullets. My young mind frantically tried to keep up with the proceedings and provide answers to the court. My voice was quiet and reluctant, as the explicit details of the event were bantered around the room.

I tried desperately to hold onto the last bit of strength I could summon, but my resolve shattered when I lifted my eyes and peeked through my hair, which I had purposefully let fall in front of my face to form a physical barrier between myself and the man. His smile struck me, stinging my cheeks like I had just received a back handed slap. Tears welled in my eyes and flowed silently from the corners and streamed down my cheeks.

I stared at my mother, her face solemn. She sat stoically in the large deserted room. Our gazes met, and for an undetermined time the room became silent, still, it was just her and me. Our voiceless conversation gave me strength, I knew I had to finish this and find the courage to go on. I looked down to the floor of the box that encased me, its simple grains of wood helped focus my attention. I composed myself and answered the final uncomfortable questions, my humiliation fully exposed. I hung my head in shame and walked disgraced from the court room, my life dishonoured. I had now become an Australian statistic, a victim of crime, with no more relevance or significance to the court, or these people.

"Who will tell whether one happy moment of love or the joy of breathing or walking on a bright morning and smelling the fresh air, is not worth all the suffering and effort which life implies."

~Erich Fromm

Chapter 6

A broken mirror
> *Pain is inevitable. Suffering is optional.*
> *~M. Kathleen Casey*

I was expected to get on with my life, unmarked or disfigured by the incident. On the outside, I was able to portray a picture to others that I was coping okay, but on the inside, a wound festered and grew purposefully. My deeply buried shame was locked securely away, my sorrow manifested only in hidden, silent words that would never be expressed, and tears shed nightly into my pillow. I mentally built a castle that rose from the ashes of my life, and allowed it to surround me. It would eventually become an inflexible fortress, its walls created from all the painful memories and the footings cemented by a loss of trust in all of humanity.

My family believed life would return to some sort of normalcy, but what is normal to one, is not always normal to another. My life never did return to the way it was before, my destiny changed, my path forever altered.

I turned inwards, not allowing the world, or anyone in it, to touch me. I locked myself away and tried to confront the dark parts of myself. I tried to banish my feelings by suppressing them, putting them in what I considered to be well-sealed containers, hiding them in niches on my carefully constructed wall of emotions. However, my feelings of revulsion, self-loathing, disgust, disempowerment and shock only matured over time. My internal war battled on, a battle of mind and emotions against youthful rationality as I tried to understand: why?

I fell into an abyss of silent questioning. The daily reflection I saw in the mirror showed unfocused eyes and a void that offered no tangible answers to any of my questions. My former, carefree, respectable behaviour transformed into complete disorder and chaos, which left both my parents bewildered. My father would leave the room and my mother would look away when I entered the room. This made me feel unwanted, dirty and rejected. It was as if I had no relevance in their lives anymore.

An unspoken, mutually agreed pact had formed between us. One of withdrawal, distractions and isolation. Long, silent months passed, our lives torn apart, forever changed. Our loving family bond broken, replaced by false pretences and rituals. We were once three loving family members who were strongly bonded. Now, we were just three people, living under the same roof. In the days and months that followed, I remembered not the harsh, or soft, words of those that once loved me, but the prevailing, persistent silences.

"For if there is a sin against life, it consists perhaps not so much in despairing of life as in hoping for another life and in eluding the implacable grandeur of this life."

~Albert Camus

Chapter 7

Struggling to survive

We have no right to ask when sorrow comes, "Why did this happen to me?" unless we ask the same question for every moment of happiness that comes our way.
~Author Unknown

Looking back, I can see that major struggles are built into the nature of everyone's life. I believe we experience them to teach us significant and fundamental lessons. They help us to grow, but quite often, I wondered, why? I frequently wondered what the purpose was, especially for what I went through.

I found the greatest of my battles was not between me and another, but the conflict inside myself. The war between my feelings and my mind was sometimes especially long and intense.

Shortly after the incident occurred I found myself dealing with a very difficult situation. I don't know why, but my school was notified of what had happened. It was supposed to have been discussed in confidence. However, Chinese whispers swept through the school like a fierce cyclone and brought with them destructive, hurtful rumours and innuendos. I became the brunt of off-handed jokes, used by gossip-mongers to make themselves look good for cheap, insensitive humour. The sole outcome obviously to belittle me in the face of my adversity.

I fought and wrestled both internally and externally with these hurtful, underhandedly slung pieces of clay. That saying "sticks and stones may break my bones but names will never hurt me," this statement isn't always true. Words do have the capability to penetrate even the strongest of physical and emotional amours, especially when it has been weakened. Some of their vicious words cut me deeply, these barbed comments pierced right into my heart.

As a self-preservation tactic, I discarded most of my old behaviours. I no longer went to school early or played and socialised. I found myself simply going through the motions. My life became full of daily rituals.

At 8 years old, I had learnt to shut myself away within the safety of my castle walls, as I tried to work out what I did and didn't feel comfortable with. As the months slipped by, I slowly taught myself to be more resilient, self-reliant and tough. I did this by simply practising different techniques and assessing the best process to use to get what I wanted and needed.

After school, instead of playing, I would fool around with a homemade Ouija board, as well as a pendulum which my mother had bought for me. She dabbled a lot in the dark arts, which led me to recognise that I was quite intuitive. Seeing, talking and predicting events was a natural experience for me, even before my life changing event. So for me, using these tools to communicate with the dead was not unnatural or scary as some would imagine. It was quite normal and my mother often nurtured and promoted my obsession with these toys.

I believed I could actually communicate with the dead using these apparatuses. At times, the room would become icy cold, and I would often see hazy figures conjured up from the floor or walls, so I knew I was not alone. Over time, I taught myself to read cards, and soon after, progressed to reading tarot cards. Later in life, I would use these skills, to provide readings for people and earn some money.

"Hope is like the sun, which, as we journey toward it, casts the shadow of our burden behind us".

Samuel Smiles

Chapter 8

Peace unveiled
The robbed that smiles, steals something from the thief.
~William Shakespeare, Othello

Our family life had changed, our relationship had changed, we all knew nothing could take us back to the innocence of the past. Living in Sydney made me feel exposed and I guess it also affected my parents, as my father accepted a long-term posting to Madang in Papua New Guinea.

I was eleven, it was 1974, and I was initially traumatized and outraged at the thought of giving up my solace and safe haven, the only life I knew. However, it didn't take me long to realise that there was a possibility that the event could be eternally locked away, and I could have a chance at some sort of a normal life, away from the prying, knowing eyes of those aware of what had occurred.
Madang was everything Sydney wasn't. It was small, beautiful, unaffected by the world's boundaries or limitations. It was untamed, unregimented, and, it liberated me. I swam in its oceans teeming with colourful fish, I watched the sun set over magnificent mountain ranges, I regained my courage and stepped out and trusted a brave new world, and it altered my life in such constructive and positive ways.

This move was a welcome distraction for all of us. I noticed that the whole family started to laugh again. My brother, 4 years old when we left Sydney, initially demanded to go home, but not long after we arrived and settled, even he began to have fun. I was optimistic that this foreign country would offer a better life for me.

My first year in Madang gave me both comfort and contentment. I felt free, enlightened, satisfied with what this new life offered. I now shared my life with new, diverse, confident friends who knew nothing of my past; people who didn't judge or ridicule me. A brand new start was on offer, and I accepted it with open arms. I was liberated, my chains crushed, my former bondage and confinement terminated. I was free to enjoy this new terrain. It offered a landscape full of intrigue, glorious sun-kissed seascapes surrounded by exotic, unexplored jungle, and it beckoned for me to venture in to.

Our first home was a three bedroom house in a suburb called Yomba, on the outskirts of the tiny town. Later that first year, we moved into a larger home in the middle of town which provided easier access to local schools and services. Nothing could have been better for me. I had found happiness and freedom from the bonds of Sydney.

Living in the middle of town was wonderful. I roamed freely. I rode my push bike through the narrow, unsealed streets, galloped my horse on the local greenery and swam in the large, under-utilized resort swimming pools. Those days were happy, carefree and fun-filled.

Madang was a very social place. Drinking and partying was the common recreational activity for the adults, and my parents were no exception; they embraced this culture wholeheartedly. As time passed, the bouts of heavy drinking increased, as did the physical altercations between my parents. During these inebriated, aggressive fights, I would either retreat to my bedroom, or scamper down the stairs to grab my bike, sprinting off and riding unnoticed through the deserted night streets.

As an adult, looking back through the eyes and experience of my 48 years, I now understand that the torment my parents felt and the frustration over the past events held them prisoners in their own self-conflict. Conflict they had no skill to resolve. Me, I was a living, breathing, constant reminder of what happened in Sydney. Alcohol, and a move, was only a temporary band-aid for a much deeper wound.

I believe, my mother felt guilt and responsibility for sending me to the shop; a guilt she would never discuss. It was, however, a guilt she would wear daily, and one that would stay with her and settle in her heart. My dad outwardly displayed himself as an unemotional man, yet, in reality he is governed by his emotions, his passion, his anger and his concern for others. This situation brought all of those emotions bubbling to the surface. Both of them were affected by the event, we were all just affected in different ways.

Philosophers say, the keys to happiness include a short memory, as well as living so that our memories will be part of our happiness. Madang was helping me learn how to focus on the good things and not dwell on all the bad. I knew I was succeeding, because the dark passenger within me didn't rise up and try to consume me as much as it did before.

"We mourn the transitory things and fret under the yoke of the immutable ones."

~Paul Eldridge

Chapter 9

Tranquillity transformed

"When written in Chinese the word "crisis" is composed of two characters - one represents danger and the other represents opportunity".
~John F. Kennedy, address, 12 April 1959

Madang offered me a life like a field of dreams. Nothing was to be feared, just explored and understood. I was able to create new circumstances. Flowers grew out of all of the dark moments I previously witnessed. The native Bougainvilleas randomly attached and flowered against the fortress walls I had previously built to protect myself.

Madang taught me not to fear life or be afraid anymore. It showed me how to live again. It taught me that storms in life come and go, and that all seas can be navigated by a skilled captain. I also realized that smooth seas do not always make skilful sailors. I leant that it is the turbulent times in life that bring forth the skills needed for the future. Madang also taught me how to appreciate my surroundings, and to see the beauty in the moment, and I was a quick learner.

Unfortunately, the tranquility and peace that surrounded me during those first years in Madang faded. Schooling opportunities for higher grades in PNG were limited to either home schooling, requiring parental guidance and input, attending the local high school with a limited program, or, choice number three, boarding school in Australia.

My parents of twelve years chose number three, thinking they were providing the best education for me. So, I was sent back to Australia, alone. A new path was chosen for me. A strict boarding school was where I was headed. A place where I would spend the next four years of my life alone, without my family and the life that could have made me whole again.

In hindsight, if only my parents had chosen to keep their fragile, damaged, teenage daughter together in the family unit, and let the nurturing, healing environment she was thriving in work its magic on her ..... if only they had disregarded formal education standards and pressures in lieu of my emotional security, then I may not have found myself writing this book.

To say I felt devastated, rejected, mentally flung back onto the ground of that damp cemetery ground would understate my feelings. Being hurt, abandoned by the people I loved the most, left a huge hole in my heart, one I didn't know how to heal. All that Madang had taught me, now, lost in the chasms of a dark, unending pit. Sydney and all its previously smothered feelings slowly bubbled to the surface, awakening the sleeping volcano within me. Scorching flames licked constantly at my wounds, reopening them. A cloud of ash surrounded me, my visibility now inadequate to see any hope; my future as bleak as the skies above me.

Adversity is a fact of life; I understood that. I had lived enough of it already. I couldn't control it. What I could control was me, and I just needed to discover how I was to fit and react to this new difficulty. I was alone in a far-off land. Unfamiliar surroundings, unknown rituals, strangers with their own foreboding troubles bordered me. There was no escape. I yearned for the family, and the short life I had grown to trust. Madang beckoned me, reached out for me in every breathe I took, but, I knew I could not allow myself to listen. So, I muted my hearing and allowed the shadows to hide my vision of the field of dreams I thought at one time could dominate my life.

I didn't want to start a new life. I was not ready for this journey. I was just a lone, terrified, young cub in need of family support. Instead, I found myself in a harsh environment, about to face a bleak extended winter on the freezing plains, alone and surrounded by a tribe of unknown hunters all carrying their own battle scars. Boarding school proved to be a desolate, ice covered rocky plain, inhospitable, unfriendly, isolated and confining. At first I didn't know how to act or behave. The arctic base, which was now my home, was governed by autocratic foreigners, exercising absolute power and extensive rules and regulations. Expectations were high.

Expectations I would never fulfil, but would quickly learn to circumnavigate.

Living under a stringent regime was hard for me. I rebelled frequently. Freedom from this harsh new setting was my only option. I knew to survive I needed to plan my escape, even if it only lived in my flamboyant imagination.

I was not the only person who suffered from family rejection. Young girls like me - children, really - surrounded me, dozens of them. All of us initially shocked to find ourselves alone, amongst unfamiliar people. We were all foreigners in a new land, aliens, testing the terrain to see just how hospitable it would be.

My second night was just as bleak and lonely as the first. As I lay face up on my single cot, I reflected on my situation, and I heard whispered cries of emotional pain beside me. Silently, I reached over and grabbed her hand to offer comfort. I listened to her choking sobs and slow, sorrowful gulps as she mourned the loss of her life. I truly felt her pain, and knew that I was not alone in my suffering, yet my own circumstances and self-preservation reactions prevented me from sharing that pain with her or anyone else, for fear of exposing my own vulnerabilities further in my lonely, cold and bitter world.

> *"God asks no man whether he will accept life. That is not the choice. You must take it. The only question is how."*
>
> *~Henry Ward Beecher*

Chapter 10

A Chameleon's life

Adversity introduces a man to himself.
~Author Unknown

Many people shared this arctic base with me, most shrouded by their own internal conflicts and unrest. Some of us joined and formed a friendship, whilst others were left to their own restlessness. However, I held to my belief that I could not rely on anyone else. I viewed my captors and their schedules as a reliable, known enemy, which was more preferable than my unpredictable family, who had discarded me.

I did form alliances, but my personal motto stood firm within me. I would do it alone, as I would not allow myself to be broken by anyone. The walls of my protective castle, now again devoid of flowers and bougainvilleas, entirely erected, fortified. I was now bordered and protected from the outside physical hurts of the world, able to combat the bitter, cold wind that internally blew and threatened to destroy my carefully constructed existence.

Over time I perfected the art of wearing two faces. Like the joker, my painted face adapted to fit into whatever circumstances I found myself in. Only I was privy to the authentic person being moulded as I grew in this sterile, unaffectionate environment.

As monotonous schedules slowly ticked by, I vowed no one would ever get close enough to me ever again. This included my family. This same family that abandoned me, left me to rot in this prison whilst they amused themselves with family holidays and excitement in exotic tropical locations. Was this a decent and fitting punishment for me after the event that happened? I thought it was a bit extreme, but I was powerless and incapable to change my current situation. I swore that when I was older, I would never feel disempowered ever again, and I would never lose control of my situation.
My outer shell portrayed a tough, resilient, hardened, young woman, however, inside I was just a teenager with emotional issues who needed guidance, love and acceptance.

Chapter 11

Reflection on my life

Looking back, I think my life would have been vastly different if someone had taken the time to really get to know me, understand the hidden pain of that event, the trauma it caused and the self-destruction it brought upon me. But it didn't happen, and I was left to fend for myself; a bird with a broken wing. There was no counselling, no psychotherapy and no recognition of post-traumatic stress. No one had a splint for my broken wing.

I could have reached out and touched the lives of the other lost girls in that boarding school. Maybe even had some lifelong friends, but I didn't. Instead, I closed myself off, not allowing anyone to get anywhere near me. I simply entered what I call survival mode.

Reflection is a wonderful thing. Over the years, I have come to recognise that whatever struggle lies before you, you must continue to move forward; the summit and all it holds may only be one step away. At the time, I refused to give things a positive go. Instead, I chose to shut myself off from situations and relationships. I also gave up far too soon in most of my life situations, regretfully not reaching my full potential or having the opportunity to unravel the secrets life was holding for me.

"Nothing great was ever achieved without enthusiasm."

Ralph Waldo Emerson

Chapter 12

Broken bonds

"Family quarrels are bitter things. They don't go by any rules. They're not like aches or wounds; they're more like splits in the skin that won't heal because there's not enough material."
~*F. Scott Fitzgerald*

My negative, internal self-talk dominated my life. It drowned me with destructive pounding waves, dragged me to the bottom and pinned me to the jagged coral below as it tore at my skin. It completely overpowered my aspirations and confidence in any form of a positive future. I continually faced self-imposed obstacles, which prevented me from pursuing any of the values and dreams that Madang had once held for me.

I forfeited the development of positive social skills and chasing happiness and love to become a skilled, sole survivor. I may have had the opportunity to become a jovial woman who understood the boundaries of love and embraced a positive desire to explore the world and make something of herself, but I would never know. Instead, I focused on regimented behaviour, containment, isolation and rejection. I chose to survive the ride and that became my only interest. I knew I would be free soon, counting down the days, 1,460 to be exact. A long time for anyone to be absent from a family, and many things change in that timeframe.

I visited my family during the school holiday, but our relationship was never the same. It was now burnt, scorched by the blistering flames of a rejection, loneliness, bitterness and time. They say absence makes the heart grow fonder; I didn't find that at all. To me, my absence from the family unit destroyed my love like water does to fire.

My love for my family changed. I no longer felt the same way about them. I had changed. My heart had hardened and a distinct barrier grew between us. I have heard it said that the love that burns the brightest leaves the deepest scars, how very true. My family's abandonment and rejection of me left deep marks upon my skin,

blemishes that couldn't be easily erased. I had loved them deeply once, but now I dared not venture into that territory again.
I had grown so independent, so manipulative and intolerant, that I no longer blended with my family values, which made it virtually impossible to merge with this group of people during my visits. I found myself constantly in trouble, unable and unwilling to conform to the family system, and the set of laws that applied to their world. I was not a part of their world any longer; they had alienated me, separating me from this unit by choice. Trying to enforce their laws upon me only resulted in frequent angry outbursts and sometimes extreme punishment.

Fights and disagreements became my normal cycle. I no longer cared how they perceived me. Boarding school taught me how to suppress my emotions, especially my feelings and how not to reveal them. So, when I came home I threw caution to the wind, as I had nothing to lose. I believed that mulling over issues such as how much my behaviour affected them was providing a small thing a big shadow and I wasn't prepared to ruin my holiday with stuff like that.

My parents were so disgusted in my behaviour and attitude that neither of them made any effort to understand me or bothered to spend any time with me. Neither of them realised that their actions had contributed to this outcome, and most of the time I was left to my own devices. Furthermore, neither of them would come to the airport to say goodbye as I returned to school in Australia. I sometimes wondered why they bothered to bring me home at all.

If only they had tried a different tactic, one that demonstrated tenderness, affection or one of friendship and acceptance, maybe the situation could have been very different. Neither of us tried any constructive avenues to reignite the fire of our relationship. We allowed our doubts and uncertainties to rob our family of any potential benefits that we may have discovered if either of us had only attempted to rebuild a relationship.

> *"The art of life is the art of avoiding pain."*
>
> *~Thomas Jefferson*

Chapter 13

Daunting scenario
"For lack of an occasional expression of love, a relationship strong at the seams can wear thin in the middle".
~Robert Brault

Four years passed, my parentally-financed and -imposed solitary confinement period finally over, my sentence finished, completed. I had earned my parole, now to be released from my jailors back to the custody of strangers. My release was pending the arrival of my estranged family, an imminent reunion with people who I shared a history with, but nothing else. A new town. This time, Rockhampton was to be my home, and I was never to see my sanctuary Madang ever again. All its hope and prospect floating in the wind, forever lost, drifting a long way from Rockhampton.

The life I had created, my solitary and autonomous life of the last four years, was about to be altered again. I was now entitled to live in a family unit again, with three other people I hardly knew. I believed I had good reason for apprehension and dread, our past turbulent histories firmly and vividly recorded on the deck of my ship. I didn't require any illustration to recall the crashing seas and isolation I felt every holiday.

I felt external silent expectations on me to be happy. I should be happy to move to another city. I should be happy to be enrolled in another school. I should be happy to take my list of fellow boarding school comrades and peers back to zero. The truth was, I was more nervous and filled with angst rather than happiness.

My previous holiday experiences marred any foreseen positives, including being positively accepted. I was seen as just the troublemaker who came home to visit every now and then, and yes, I got into quite a lot of mischief. I smoked my first joint, drunk alcohol, attended all night parties, had my first sexual experience and tried the local beetle nut all whilst on holiday from school.

I wasn't excited; I was scared. I tried to imagine what it would be like sharing a house, not a dorm, having my own private space, and a bathroom only four people used, instead of twenty. It was a foreign concept after living in close proximity in a dormitory that overflowed with girls, yet, I welcomed the freedom it offered from the rules, tyrants and my current captors.

My family scared me. I knew nothing about them and they knew nothing, really, about me. Years had passed. I left when I was twelve, now I was sixteen, my youth stolen in the prison of academia. I emerged transformed, altered by what I had experienced. I embraced new skills not formerly known in my life in Madang.

Physically and mentally, I was tougher, hardened by my sufferings. To survive boarding school, I had locked myself away in a sealed castle of selfishness, embracing a hardened spirit and mind. My heart was impenetrable and irredeemable. How could I live with these people again? I had lived so long locked away inside myself, I was unsure if it was even possible to share my life with anyone.

My outside facade portrayed a tough exterior, a poor representation of what was really happening on the inside. I was anxious about this move. I didn't recall any positive experiences regarding the whole family situation, and the family concept was unfamiliar, foreign to me. How would I transition from my safe autonomous bubble currently protecting me, to a life that involved three other people?

What were their expectations of me now? I obviously had not acted the way they had wanted when I visited, so I had absolutely no idea how to act now. A chameleon needs to assess and understand the situation before it can appropriately change its colours. It would take me a few weeks before I could change my form to fit in enough to survive. The same feelings I experienced that first week at boarding school revisited me, unleashing apprehension and anxiety. A sense of dread set fire to any optimism I felt I would just have to figure it out by trial and error.

The day arrived. They picked me up, smiling. It was an awkward moment as we embraced, hugged and kissed. Small, inconsequential dialogue lapsed between us, as we drove off to a new beginning.

Chapter 14

Lost in a changing world
Sometimes it is the person closest to us who must travel the furthest distance to be our friend.
*~**Robert Brault***

It appeared to me that during my absence, my parents and my brother had formed a strong three-corded, loving bond. Laughter filled the air as they revealed experiences that I had no part in, holidays they shared and friends they encountered and missed.

Affection was also an unfamiliar exchange. I had forgotten what it was like to be cuddled or touched, and I was uncomfortable watching the three of them trade affection in this manner.
In the early days of separation from my family, I would crave affection and any sort of attention. I would lie in my single bunk, facing my whole world, which was encased in one small cupboard, and quietly cry myself to sleep. Abandonment deeply distorts and somehow taints the nature of a person. Those nights changed my character, especially as I listened all around me as the soft sobs echoed across the bleak walls of the long dormitory room. Our beds were close enough that when I extended my arm, I could touch the next person, so I would reach out and gently stroke the back of the girl next to me providing comfort and solace to her.

It was at this moment I realize just how much we all needed to feel some sort of affection. A simple act of an innocent and gentle touch gave us hope in the unfamiliar world. It enabled us to cope with our estrangement from the familiar world of families that were ripped from us. This was the last real affection I felt or knew, and to now see people openly cuddling each other was beyond my understanding.

I didn't realise that this was normal for people who lived together. It certainly was not normal from the experiences that were a part of my life. I again struggled not knowing how to merge into this cosy circle. I didn't feel comfortable being a part of it, and, I didn't feel really welcomed or embraced by it either. I sensed this unit was quite wary of me as well, keeping me at a distance, exposing me only to the necessary sections of their lives.

My brother, now aged 9, was much more fascinating. He was significantly more interesting than my previous holiday visits, where he just annoyed me. I was drawn to his amusing and extremely comical nature. He was spirited and made me laugh enthusiastically until pains in my stomach prevented me from continuing. We spent a lot of time together as we resurrected a relationship that should have been naturally present.

On weekends, we would walk to the local council-owned pool. We swam, surrounded by other snotty-nosed children, and ate frozen ice blocks until we got a brain freeze. We played the old pin ball machines and fought over the Kiss machine and Space Invaders game. We battled and we laughed and taunted each other until it was time to go home.

My brother was cute and his laugh infectious. Often, his antics and games made me roll on the bed in hysterics. He was quite the show man, wanting to be a clown and a magician when he grew up. I thought this was hilarious. Not that he wasn't talented, it just didn't seem to me to be a great career choice.

It didn't take long for me to learn to love this kid again; he didn't judge or condemn me, he actually thought I was cool, and he brought a smile to my lips when I thought of him. I was important in his life and I liked that.

"The true harvest of my daily life is somewhat as intangible and indescribable as the tints of morning or evening. It is a little star dust caught, a segment of the rainbow which I have clutched."

~Henry David Thoreau, Walden

Chapter 15

A time to yield

You can kiss your family and friends good-bye and put miles between you, but at the same time you carry them with you in your heart, your mind, your stomach, because you do not just live in a world but a world lives in you.
~Frederick Buechner

My life, it seemed, had established itself into some sort of routine, a stable pattern that I could understand and manage. Dad had purchased a new house, I was reasonably settled into a new school and had met some interesting people. I thought we had found a sustainable rhythm that was comfortable for everyone.

However, shortly after we moved into our new home, my mother chose to return to Sydney for a visit. This was not unusual for her as she was a travel agent and travelled extensively. On one occasion, I arrived home from boarding school for one of my short visits to find my mother embarking on a personal holiday to Sydney; she would be gone the whole time I was there. Her departure at the time just fuelled my internal fire of rejection.

My parent's actions, attitudes and behaviour towards me on all my visits cut deep. It wounded me, leaving profound scars both mentally and physically. I now believe, one of the greatest gifts you can give to someone is the honour of your attention. However, I didn't receive that from my family, especially my mother. My mother's constant spiteful words hurt my feelings, but her silences broke my heart. She made me feel unwelcomed, unloved and very unimportant in her life. So when she informed me she was going to Sydney once again, it meant very little to me, as I had already become accustomed to this sort of rejection.

Being away for so long made me a stranger in their world; this four year absence prevented me from being able to discern any threatening undercurrents that could potentially de-stabilise the family unit. Their behaviours and routines were unfamiliar to me, so I was unable to read the little signs of unhappiness, bitterness and poor communication. From my limited perspective, things looked pretty normal, okay. These parents might have been my blood, but I was blind-folded and handicapped when it came to understanding their world.

Despite what was going on around us, my brother and I continued to build our repertoires of dreams. We collected and collated memories, and catalogued shared experiences as we made up for lost time. Both of us naive to our environment and the trouble brewing, we lived in a dreamscape full of promises. Neither of us suspected the dark cloud looming overhead would separate our worlds with its lightening strike.

I didn't have much time or inclination to worry about my mother's intentions. I had my own daily struggles and integration process to worry about. My new school held lots of conflict. I have come to know that there are two ways of dealing with difficulties: you either alter the challenge or you alter yourself to rise up and meet it head on. You can fight the adversity or fight yourself, both create changes and both have a place in life.

I chose to fight my adversity, school was becoming quite a problem, and I knew I needed to fight for some sort of acceptance. This offered a huge challenge for me. I had to risk going too far, to discover just how far I could really go in gaining some form of acceptance. I had a strategy which worked in part, and it certainly drew a lot of attention, especially from the show pony girls and the misfit boys.

My first act was to blatantly refuse to wear the short, blue uniform, choosing instead to wear a floor length navy skirt and un-ironed blouse. The second act was to show my rebellious nature, that old coat that I wore in previous times. I knew that it alone would attract a lot of trouble. It was easy. I slipped on my well-worn, familiar coat and waited for their reactions.

They came thick and fast. Firstly the teachers wanted me to explain my choice of clothing, and my behaviour. Well, detention became my second home and "wagging" school became a weekly occurrence. I also caught the eye of a very good looking young man, tall, athletic, blonde-haired, brown-eyed surfer, all of which is another story. I will say we were together for some time and then hooked up again a few years later but, no, it didn't work out.

Uneventful days slipped into weeks, and my mother still hadn't returned from Sydney. This scenario left my father in a state of mild panic, as he tried to care for two children as well as working fulltime. Curiosity was getting the better of me; where was she? What was taking her so long? Why had she not made any contact with any of us?

And one day, soon after I had pondered these questions my reply came.

It came one day as I sat in a quiet classroom with 25 other single-minded, distracted teenagers. My pencil drew circles and lines in non-descript patterns on my spiral-bound book. Suddenly, my concentration was interrupted; I heard my name called by the teacher demanding my attention. I looked up, and was shocked to see my dad as he stood outside the classroom door, waiting for me.

Inquisitive eyes focused on me from around the room. I slowly rose from my hard plastic seat, embarrassment swept over me, yet I was curious why he was here. I gathered my books into a large pile and placed them in my oversized bag and shoved the rest of my belongings into the side pouch. Then I slowly shuffled to the door. I tried not to draw any more attention to myself, however, I knew it was too late for that. Questioning eyes tracked my every move, hungry for any ounce of gossip. I had been the brunt of malicious gossip once before, and it left a foul taste in my mouth, so I would not give them anything to talk about if I could help it.

My father stood impatiently at the door. However, when I saw him, I realized that what I thought was impatience was actually distress. His red, puffy eyes held suppressed tears as they patiently waited for the right moment to be released. What did this mean? He toyed with his hands and pulled slightly at his collar, something serious had happened, otherwise he wouldn't be here. My mind started creating scenes of chaos. Visions of my brother being injured in an accident at school, now in a hospital bed seriously injured. NO, a voice screamed within me, not him, he was my ally, the only bright shiny star I had.

I was jolted from these images, by a thin rectangular object as it was thrust into my hand. I dragged my eyes away from my father's face and all that it held, to look down at a small white envelope, addressed to me. I noticed my mother's handwriting scribbled on the surface. The tattered outer edges of the letter caught my attention. It had been opened. It was then that I realized my father had already read its contents, and the penny dropped.

I looked from my father to the letter and back again. Finally, I opened it and read the dark script written delicately upon the paper, words that carried a heavy burden. A simple letter, with simple words, not very emotive, more matter of fact. It straightforwardly informed me of her intentions to stay in Sydney, and contained a frank statement about not being able to take either my brother or myself at this time. She asked if I would look after him, and then it ended with her regret and sadness. Whoa...... Okay, I didn't see that coming!

Unanswered questions shrieked at me. Why me? Why tell me this news? In a letter, of all things! Why had she not rung to tell us in person? Why address it to me? It should have been addressed to dad. It concerned him more than me. I didn't understand her actions at all. What did she expect of me? I knew I was not in any emotional place, where I was capable of doing anything positive with this family.

Look after my brother. Now, that was a big ask. What could I do? What parenting skills did I possess? Absolutely none. I couldn't be his role model, I was too dysfunctional and carried far too many wounds that hadn't had time to heal.

I wondered if this was what all families were like. Nothing ever seemed to run smoothly. One minute, things seemed okay, and the next, everything was shattered. No wonder kids run away, and for a split second, I considered it; living my own life far away from all this drama would be great. However, the desperation, pain and suffering I witnessed on my father's face, and the newly found love for my brother held me back.

Laurie Smyth

Question after question cycled through my brain. Was this really happening? I kept asking why, why? Was this happening because I was now home? Was I that bad and unlovable that my presence could cause this sort of reaction? Did she despise me that much that she resorted to this kind of reaction?

"In life, as in restaurants, we swallow a lot of indigestible stuff just because it comes with the dinner."

~Mignon McLaughlin, The Neurotic's Notebook, 1960

Chapter 16

Mourning a lost dream
"To be lost in life is to keep your mind, eyes, and ears covered."
Byron Pulsifer

I realised that if we were to go through life without any obstacles, we would be mentally crippled, not growing as we are meant to.
My dad really struggled to fight this war on his own. The combat at times overpowered him, incapacitated him. His lone campaign to maintain the empire he had built for all of us to share, as well as trying to sustain my brother and I, quickly took its toll on him, and it crumbled around us. He was forced to sell our beautiful home and rent a small, two bedroom, bottom-floor flat on a main street. He endeavoured to overcome his emotional wounds and rebuild our broken family, but his rotational roster and the enforced second job he required to make ends meet left me and my brother alone for long periods of time.

During these long lonely months, we drew on each other's strength. We forged a close connection, and an uncomplicated bond of need developed between us. It nurtured and healed us. At night I would lay beside him as he snuggled underneath the covers. I would lay on top of his doona and stroke his hair, hoping to provide him some comfort. His tears broke my heart; I knew I could never take away his pain. A horrid stillness descended upon his life. The loss of his mother, his feelings of abandonment and the disintegration of his dreams and expectations was not something that could be replaced easily. It was a gap I couldn't possibly fill.

The rain would come, and I would walk and walk and walk, allowing the drizzle to splatter on my face, so it could disguise my many tears. My brother's anguish cut deeper than any other sorrow I had felt. No human being can really understand another's pain and suffering, and I could only put bandages on the wounds I saw. I only hoped that his scars would not run as deep as mine. I would spare him that if I could. My feelings were not as intense as his. My connection with my mother was not as deep. But, if I could have changed the circumstances for him, I would have done just about anything.

My demons started to surface again, as feelings of responsibility emerged. Shadowy voices blamed me for the whole bleak scenario. They reminded me that I had just returned to the family, and now it was torn apart, so soon after my return. It was obviously my fault. Guilt rose like the forthcoming dawn. It's blaze flaunted words of torment and blame at me; its goal, to destroy my self-esteem further. We were simply two broken kids, one more damaged than the other. We sought to find our way out of the maze our lives had been dumped in, as well as attempt to somehow rebuild our shattered lives.

> *"Believe with all of your heart that you will do what you were made to do."*
>
> ***Orison Swett Marden***

Chapter 17

Life burst into flames

"The price of anything is the amount of life you exchange for it."
*~**Henry David Thoreau***

Time takes our expectations, hopes and dreams with it and places them behind us in the past. Then the past gently rolls away out of our reach as the future unravels before us. Time slipped quietly, mostly unnoticed, away from us, but it brought development into our new family unit. We found mutual harmony and a peaceful reality in our new life roles. Happiness was yet to return, but we reawakened the laughter which had lain dormant within each of us. Months went by, which enabled us to plant some seeds, with the hope that they would grow and mature within each of us into something positive.

Out of the blue, my mother commenced contact with myself and my brother. This new situation caused major unrest and instability in our currently stable unit. As she continued to converse with my brother and I through letters and phone conversations, we felt torn between theW life we had built and the life she now promised.

My parent's relationship had deteriorated to the state of divorce; how it got there, I don't know, as I was not privy to any of their conversations. I do know that she continually threatened my father with custody, and this took its toll on him. Torment and distress compelled him to consider his options to provide what he thought was a better home for us. His view on a more stable, better life included another woman, who eventually moved in to our small home with her two kids. I didn't know where she came from, one day it was the three of us and the next day it was six of us. The situation took me by surprise and was very strange and extremely unsettling.

To accommodate this new family of six, dad had to buy a bigger house. I believed that he did this to keep my mother at bay. It was torture for me. I despised them being in my life; sharing a house with these foreigners was not what I had envisioned when I left boarding school. Definite but invisible boundaries now existed in our once happy home, my brother and I banded together and lines of division were clearly drawn between her children and us.

A catastrophic storm brewed in this new environment. In its wake would lay deep caverns, filled with disastrous outcomes none of us would fully recover from for a long time to come. I discovered the true meaning of betrayal. My mother had abandoned us, and now this! This move annihilated everything we had previously built in our new family unit, my brother and I now solidly bound in a pact of survival against new odds.

My father wore a cheerful, obliging disposition, his unfeigned feelings placed carefully in a bubble. Daily, he battled his emotions and rationale as he tried to seek unsought answers way beyond the obvious. If he had only noticed what was before him; the potential possibilities! But he didn't. He chose to live a lie with a woman who meant very little to him.

I witnessed his agitation, anxiety and his dread as it grew daily. He was losing his grip on his primary goal: to keep our family unit together. With his limited experience, he considered this to be the best option, a partnership purely based on necessity, and we all knew it.

One morning my father intercepted a call from my mother, who was coercing my brother over to her cause to reunite herself with her only son. Not a hard task under the circumstances we were in at the moment. Both of us hated the situation of sharing a house with these people, so my mother's option did tempt him, although her appeals fell on my deaf ears. I was attempting to undertake my Year 11 studies with a hope of re-establishing some of my lost dreams, and was not about to budge.

I was in the bathroom brushing my teeth when my father stormed in, his face red and angry. He looked like he was going to explode, his body shook uncontrollably with rage. He frightened me. His loud, fiery voice hurled accusations of my betrayal and conspiracy, all unknown to me. The sound of his tense expressions rang loudly in my ears, his words swirled around the tiny, enclosed room. He could not be reasoned with in these situations, so I refused to answer his allegations. I tried to remain calm, but I had witnessed this behaviour before, and I could feel the waves of hot flushes of panic and dread as they swept over me. I was backed into a corner, and I knew I had nowhere to go. The bathroom had only one door and he stood in it. I refused to answer, which added fuel to his fire, and suddenly he reached out and punched me.

I stepped into the bath and hunched into the corner as I tried to get away from him. My screams alerted my brother, who ran bravely to my aid, but he was just a boy. He stood in the doorway and cried and pleaded for our father to stop, and he finally did.

I grabbed my bag and ran up the hill to my school. The school that had made me believe that I could do something with my life, maybe even go onto uni and become the lawyer I dreamt of becoming. I didn't know where else to go. My heart beat strong and fast in my chest as the adrenalin pumped around my body. My legs didn't feel the hard ascending bitumen as they sprinted towards my haven.

As I reached the looming gates, I slowed my pace to a brisk walk. I didn't stop to speak to anyone, ignoring the welcoming comments, going instead straight into the cold, dark classroom. I could hide there for a few moments and gather my thoughts. I knew I had at least 20 minutes before the classes started, so I could prepare myself; pull myself together before anyone else arrived.

I didn't notice her as she watched me in the dim light. A tall, good looking women with gentle eyes stood holding an armful of books ready to be moved to the oversized wooden bookshelves. I felt her stare as it swept over me. I felt awkward and shamed under the intensity of her eyes. I needed time to think. As she briefly turned to place the books down, I looked down at my self to cover up the embarrassment that I felt. It was then that I realised my school shirt was ripped. I was horrified. I quickly picked up my bag and hugged it close to my chest. Was I quick enough? Did she see my humiliation? She slowly turned to face me, and I could see that she comprehended the indignity I felt.

I hardly heard the words that fell from her pink stained lips. I knew what she wanted to know, but I couldn't find the right words to answer her. For an extended moment our eyes shared a deep veiled conversation; she discerned the truth. I turned and walked out of school, never to return.

I spent the rest of the day wandering through the Botanical Gardens as I fantasised and contemplated a healthier, more positive life. What would it look like if my parents had stayed together? If I had not been sent away? If I had not been raped? What would my life be like without all that tragedy? Surely other families experience blissful lives with no serious adversity, or does everyone have this level of drama in their life? I wondered what happiness really looked like. What was it like to having a loving, stable family?

I understood sadness, rejection and pain, but what about the tenderness of love, trust and compassion? To feel someone reach out and touch you in love must be a beautiful sensation. Would I ever feel something like that?

The sun dipped in the sky and the warmth oozed from the day. I knew it was time for me to return home. It was around 4.30pm when I reached my house. My angry father and his uncaring girlfriend stood on the front wooden balcony, watching me as I walked up the driveway. He started yelling at me again, unfounded accusations regarding my mother fell from his lips.

He lifted a bundle of garments up in his arms and threw them over the balcony. Unmistakably, they were items that belonged to me. I watched them as they fell to the ground, sprawling across the driveway. I started slowly to pick them up as my mind processed what had occurred. I knew where this would go. Then he spoke the words I knew would come. I was sixteen and had been reunited with my family for all of eight months.

> *"Life is easier than you'd think; all that is necessary is to accept the impossible, do without the indispensable, and bear the intolerable."*
>
> *~Kathleen Norris*

Chapter 18

Cast away
"You have come into a hard world. I know of only one easy place in it, and that is the grave."
~Henry Ward Beecher

I was terrified. What was I to do? Where was I to go? Yet at the same time, I also felt liberated, free from that situation. My heart longed to reach out and touch the boy who stood crying on the veranda, my solace, my friend, my brother. Here I was once again being ripped away from someone I truly and deeply loved. I looked intensely into his face, searching for the right words. There was so much I wanted to say to him, but the words would not come. I longed to cry out to him, to tell him I loved him and things would be okay, but I remained silent, unable to express what I desperately wanted to say. I didn't know when or if I would see him again, this beautiful lost boy I had just got to know again.

It was just him and dad now against the new trespassers. I knew the relationship with this other family was temporary. I could see the unhappiness, discontent and misery that my father felt, for this situation was born out of hardship and purpose only, not based on love or desire. My mother had a lot to answer for, and as I searched my brother's eyes, and committed his face to memory, I felt the abandonment and the rejection that he suffered, and I felt real distaste for the person who bore me. She was an unpredictable ally, someone who I would use over the next few months to restore my life, but someone I would not trust again for quite some time.

I gathered the few articles of clothing that represented my life and walked out of my dad's life for a very long time.

An opportunity presented itself to move in with my boyfriend's family, and I took it. I lived in a caravan in their front yard for the next few months until I could find a unit and fulltime employment. During this time, I maintained a secret relationship with my brother. He would sneak out to meet me whilst our father worked. We would often walk down to the local café, eat burgers and talk. I missed his presence and the joy he brought into my life.

My parent's rejection caused me to become bitter, cynical and lost. I felt the world owed me and my spirit hardened towards everyone and everything, except my brother. He could melt my heart with his glance and especially his tears. I would hold him as I tried to soothe and encourage him. I knew the pain he lived with, and knew that there would be ramifications and changes in his life from this experience and anguish. I only hoped this experience would not break him like it had broken me.

Within months of leaving, my brother moved to Brisbane to be with my mother, and I lost any association and relationship to a reasonable, loving connection. A complete tragedy, all our lives devastated and the family unit shattered. My father's relationship didn't last. Neither did mine. We were both damaged and without hope.

> *"There are things known, and there are things unknown. And in between are the doors."*
>
> *- Jim Morrison*

Chapter 19

Shaking the foundations
"When it is dark enough, you can see the stars."
~Ralph Waldo Emerson

Two months short of my 17th birthday I met and moved in with a self-employed, 21-year-old business man. I was infatuated with him. He made me feel special. He filled the darkened, icy crevices of my being with his loving words and his caring actions. I was in love. I finally felt important to someone. Our lives intertwined. We created a passionate connection.

Two years into our relationship, cracks started to form and I realised I had chosen a person who could never make me feel good about myself. He was as damaged as I was; he just chose to obscure and mask his problems with excessive drinking and substance misuse. What I did was trade my previous, unemotional, non-functional life and adopted his, only to find his was more dysfunctional than mine. His appalling temper surfaced, followed by intense feelings of remorse, exacerbated by long periods of excessive drinking which led to violent altercations, more substance use and the cycle continued.

Identifying this reality made me feel more worthless and inadequate than ever before. I believed I deserved what he dished out, and that I would never amount to anything in life. His derogative words and hurtful statements only confirmed my fears. I felt trapped in this life, unable to change it, not knowing how. Our life continued, both of us unwilling to change the destructive behaviours that dominated our life together, drugs and alcohol as well as the party scene governed both of us.

I now found my life with him depressing, monotonous and pointless. When we were together, our daily life focused around bottles of Captain Morgan Rum, a few joints and listening to the harmonious melodies of Dire Straits. Smoking marijuana led me to experiment with other more exciting drugs; a progression I considered normal. Drugs were a big part of our relationship. We had tried everything on the market, at that time, acid, coke, speed, pills and marijuana were staples in our lives. However, I didn't really like acid. My first acid experience frightened me, it was full of hallucinations and rising demons, coke was my favourite and often used. Speed just made my insides rattle and my brain accelerate. Thoughts processed so fast I couldn't grasp many of them, and marijuana made me so mellow and eat far too much.

At nineteen, drugs were accepted and fully utilised parts of my daily existence. I found myself drawn into a taboo culture, one I thought I would never enter. Heroin beckoned me. It fascinated me. Some of the people we socialised with were regular users. They were different from our other friends. Nothing seemed to faze them, living a peaceful life, yet also quite functional, working and some were parents, but they were continually broke. They interested me. The whole scene appealed to me. It was a forbidden product, a societal no-no, and heroin users were considered outlaws who lived an unaccepted lifestyle concealed from the law. Their lifestyles full of risk, unknown hazards and danger, it fascinated me! My first experience was the best escape I had ever indulged in, better than anything I had tried before. Certainly better than the "mull" we smoked, this had substance to it. I would regularly indulge in using these drugs to allow them to blanket my turbulent life with its calming affects.

I never believed that I could actually put the tip of a sharp needle on my vein and stick it in. But, when the time came and the needle penetrated my arm, my blood swirled and mixed with the clear solution, then retreated down to the tip to enter my body, I was not thinking of any of those decisions. As a young child, I had so many dreams and aspirations; plans I wanted to achieve when I was finally an adult. None occurred to me at that moment and none awaited me now.

By the age of nineteen, I was pregnant. I was happy at the concept of bringing a child into this world. I believed that becoming a mother would alter my entire situation in a positive way. I craved the concept of real love and experiencing unconditional love for the first time, and I thought that I would automatically receive that from this child. I also stupidly believed that my partner and I would become that happy family unit portrayed in magazines and television - Rational thinking in a drug-induced haze at the time. However, it was a completely unrealistic expectation.

I knew that if this philosophy was to work, I would have to learn some mothering skills. A concept way beyond my reach, as my own relationship with the only role model I knew was not terribly good. So I would need to learn as I went. My mother's parenting and teaching classes finalized when I was eleven. So I had limited experience in constructive or beneficial hands on relationships. But, I knew I would give it my best shot. During my pregnancy I refused to take anything harder than marihuana and forfeited everything else, until after the birth.

And I gave birth to a beautiful English rose, my daughter Jade. I would never make mother of the year, but, I loved her more than I thought humanly possible. My love grew with every passing day. It filled me and overflowed, and still there was room for more. My bucket would never be full. I found unconditional love, but not from her; it came from inside me.

For the first time in my life I realized that the world was larger than me, that when I peered out the window, a vast landscaped awaited. My once tiny portal became a large movie screen, and important life messages were waiting for me to view them. I started to slowly take notice of what these broadcasts were saying. I sifted through and adopted some of the easier options like forfeiting some of my partying ways to be with my daughter.

My daughter was my world; her beautiful blue-green eyes filled me with a new found hope. She represented a better life. I started to see my world differently and I started to question my life. Was there a better way for me? If so, where?

My partner didn't like the constraints that parenthood brought with it, so, he spent numerous nights out drinking and partying, leaving me lost and lonely at home. My loneliness enticed me to bury my feelings in a veil of more drugs and alcohol. Our true relationship now beyond repair, hidden from view under a drug-induced coma, obscured from ourselves and the world around us. We lost ourselves and each other in a void that grew daily.

We existed like this for another two years.

I was far from living the dreams of my youth, instead I was twenty-one years old, a mother who lived in a volatile, unstable relationship, who used drugs and alcohol to self-medicate, so that I didn't have to really look at the world I had created. My dreams of going to uni shattered and gradually faded with every drug experience.

"Life is what we make it, always has been, always will be."

~Grandma Moses

Chapter 20

A precious life
"He who has a why to live can bear almost any how.
~Friedrich Nietzsche

When Jade was still a baby, I was surprised to find out that I was pregnant again. I had mixed emotions regarding this pregnancy. I loved my daughter and saw how beautiful she was, and this enticed me to have another child. But, my thoughts wandered to my behaviour, my drug use, my drinking, and I realised that I wasn't in what I would have described as the 'right head space' to have another child, not now. I knew my partner would not support me if I did decide to go through with having another child, as we had just separated again. I would have to do it alone. This prospect terrified me. I had no skills or ability to find a job that could support three people. I rationalised that my drug use could have potentially already damaged the child, and even if I stopped using now, it would be too late. So, I chose to have an abortion.

In the 1980's it was illegal to have this procedure done in Queensland. I bundled my daughter up and together we caught the train to Tweed Heads, New South Wales, where the procedure would be done.

I left my daughter with a friend, and I entered the clinic alone. I stood in front of the high counter and anxiously waited to be served. I was still unclear, and in two minds about whether or not to have the procedure. I wondered if I could I really do it. Did I really want to go through with it? I started to think about what my life would be like with two kids and no partner? How would I cope? Was it even possible? Before I could answer any of these raging questions, a nurse offered me a Valium, which I quickly swallowed. I yearned for the tranquillity and peace it would bring, and I welcomed the effects as they slowly crept over my body and stilled my busy mind.

I was taken to a sterile, white-walled surgical room, and the nurse casually prepared me for the procedure. I lay on the bed in the silence and serenity of the room and felt the full effects of the medication.

The doctor entered the room and the procedure started. I could hear the machinery as it hummed and pulsated in the background, like a hungry beast ready to devour its prey. I felt the vibrations of the instruments inside me. In my haze, I felt the baby move, its presence shocked me and I was brought back to reality and what I was actually doing. At that same moment, I thought I heard it cry out, telling me to stop. But all too soon the procedure was over and I was funnelled into a recovery area, and then sent home.

I felt that I had done the wrong thing, but it was too late and there was absolutely nothing I could do about it. The child was gone. Ripped from my body by my own doing, and I was nothing short of a murderer, and I felt like it. Even as I tried to rationalise my choice, knowing the truth that I was unable and unfit to raise another child, I still felt overwhelmed by the feelings of what I had done.

Since then, I now know what happens to the child during that process. It is literally torn apart piece by piece by the suction. Learning this made my heart ache for what I had done. I had murdered an innocent child, my own child, not someone else's, my own flesh and blood, and not by mistake, but intentionally.

Learning to forgive myself for this awful action would take many years.

> *"To preserve a man alive in the midst of so many chances and hostilities is as great a miracle as to create him".*
>
> *~Jeremy Taylor*

Chapter 21

Seeing the real world
"There is no education like adversity."
Benjamin Disraeli

Shortly after going through this procedure, I returned to my home town, but I was not the same person. A change had begun in me. I moved into a unit with another single mother and commenced work in the local night club. At the same time, my father moved to the same town I was living in and attempted to reach out to me to re-establish a relationship.

He called me without warning one day and invited me to meet him in our local hotel for some unimportant chit-chat. I can't recall what we talked about, but what I did see was just how different he had become. I witnessed a real change in him. He was more content, happier, and he carried himself differently. At the time I could not put my finger on it, but I knew he was not the angry, confused man that I left all those years ago. He had found something that made him healthier, happier and more content.

I tried to discreetly study him to ascertain the subtle changes I could see. What was it about him? He now possessed an air of self-control. One change was blatantly obvious; he had given up drinking, for he sipped lemonade. But there was more. What else had happened in his life? Something had changed and it really intrigued me. He certainly got my attention, not by our conversation, but by what I saw. We parted and he gave me a hug. I couldn't remember the last time he had embraced me in any fashion. Who was this guy? What had happened to him to change him so drastically?

As we parted, he told me he was praying for me. What a statement! I thought he was joking, but his face didn't portray that at all. He was serious. I didn't believe in any of that God stuff. Nothing good had happened in my life to make me believe in any God. I laughed at him and told him not to bother, for I was already lost and happy the way I was, but I internally pondered his statement for quite some time.

A few months passed and I grew more and more unhappy, I reconnected and disconnected from my yo-yo relationship a few more times, dabbled with other people, but nothing made me feel whole anymore.

I started to see my father quite regularly and even worked for him for a short period of time, but I grew increasingly restless and nothing in this current life fulfilled me or made me feel any real satisfaction or pleasure. I drank more, I took more drugs and I slept around more, but nothing filled the void that grew within me.

I don't know what changed in my life, but one day I looked at my beautiful young daughter as she played in the backyard and decided there must be more to life than what I was currently living. I started to consider and evaluate my life's choices. I realised that my on-again-off-again partner of five years was never going to change from his drunken path and doing drugs everyday, which would make it impossible for me to become "clean". I started to weigh up where I would be if I stayed with him. I knew I couldn't continue on this path. I could see how completely self-destructive I was. I would kill myself if nothing changed, and I was now responsible for another's life, one I would die for.

"If I had a formula for bypassing trouble, I would not pass it round. Trouble creates a capacity to handle it. I don't embrace trouble; that's as bad as treating it as an enemy. But I do say meet it as a friend, for you'll see a lot of it and had better be on speaking terms with it."

~Oliver Wendell Holmes

Chapter 22

A reawakening

"Nothing is predestined: The obstacles of your past can become the gateways that lead to new beginnings."
Ralph Blum

I decided to make a clean break. I packed up all my gear (not that I had much left, as I had sold most of it to pay for drugs and alcohol), and I took off for Townsville. I drove all day in the blazing sun, my daughter curled up in the back seat, with absolutely nowhere to go and no one I knew to help me. I had no drugs or alcohol with me. I was determined to kick my habit and change my life, and I knew I couldn't do that where everything was familiar.

When I arrived, I found a caravan park and booked and paid for a week with the only money I had, $74.00. I stayed in the van for nearly a week as I "dried out" and fought to get my life back. I can't recall what happened to my daughter during this time, but I know we were taken care of. I have no recollection as to how or who fed us or showered Jade. All I know is that we were okay during that ordeal.

After that first week I got a job as a nanny and moved in with a man and his two children, and my life moved in the right direction. A few months later, I moved into a house and got a job as a waitress and my daughter went to childcare, and life started to look up.

I started to dabble again with drugs, but not as aggressively as before. During this time, I was offered a job as a call girl and I thought, why not? I was sleeping around anyway, I may as well get paid for it. So, I did. I was earning big dollars, but a few weeks into my new found career, some money was stolen and a raid was threatened, so I packed up in the middle of the night and drove back to my hometown.

When I arrived back, everything looked different to me. My hazy glasses had been removed, revealing the true prospects of my life in this place. I wasn't the same person as when I left. I was relatively 'clean', although I still loved to drink. I noticed the scene hadn't changed, but I had, and I didn't fit anymore, and I didn't really want to. I settled down for a few months reigniting my relationship with my partner, but I really wasn't into that either. Nothing had changed, yet, everything inside of me had. My attitude and my desires were different. I wanted more from life and I was not content with living this way. I had changed more than I thought.

So, I made another choice that changed the course of my life.

"Adversity is like a strong wind. It tears away from us all but the things that cannot be torn, so that we see ourselves as we really are".

~Arthur Golden, Memoirs of a Geisha

Chapter 23

A step forward
"Every problem has in it the seeds of its own solution. If you don't have any problems, you don't get any seeds."
~Norman Vincent Peale

My relationship was over by the time I turned twenty-one, I had a two-year old child to raise, and no employment prospects. I still had a huge substance abuse problem, alcohol now my poison. I knew I couldn't stay in the same small town as my ex-lover, with all our shared friends and acquaintances. So, I moved away and traded everything I knew for a new start. This was a big decision for me, my life was based in this town. But somehow I got the courage to pack up my life, get in the car and drive in the other direction this time, to the Gold Coast.

I found the first month on this chosen path really difficult. I had initially come down to the Gold Coast as my partner's brother and his family had offered me a place to stay. I accepted their offer, but the situation became quite uncomfortable. My ex would ring and his brother would feel compelled to inform him of our movements, so I moved out to couch surf for a few weeks with a girl who had enrolled in the same Diploma of Hospitality course I was doing.

Every day I battled with the determination to go home. I questioned my resolve constantly. What sort of life was I providing for my daughter? We were living in a lounge room with no privacy, in a one bedroom flat! However, things changed quite rapidly after I moved in with her.

A week into my couch surfing experience, a two bedroom unit became vacant in the same block of flats we shared in Main beach. We took it. Around the same time, I found a really great mum to look after Jade, so I could start applying for work. All of this secured the deal for me, I decided that I was not turning back now, things were finally falling into place. I would stay and build a life for myself and my daughter on the Gold Coast. Yes, I had pangs of desire to return to my old life, but I had made a choice and I wanted to stick to it. I knew I was not yet strong enough to go back, as I knew I could easily slip back into my old habits, and that was a life I had fully turned my back on. I wanted and needed a new beginning. I wanted to build a better foundation for my daughter to grow up with.

I knew it would be tough for me to secure a real job. I had limited hospitality skills, simple basic bar skills and I was working towards obtaining a piece of paper that would hopefully help me. I could pour a beer and mix the odd drink, but working on the tourist strip on the Gold Coast was quite different than working in a small town bar. But, three weeks after arriving on the Gold Coast, I was called for an interview at a five star resort.

I had never frequented a place like that, let alone worked in anything like it. It was way above what I was used to. My local beer garden and the bar were squalid in comparison to this place, with its nine bars, three swimming pools, five eating areas, two night clubs, cocktail bar and shopping area. My knowledge about working in a resort-style environment was negligible. When I lived in Madang we would frequent a resort there for dinner and activities, but it was nothing like this one. I was exceptionally nervous about myself and my abilities in this type of position. First things first I had to get through the formal interview and that was a daunting prospect for me; this again was something I had limited experience in.

To attend, I wore the only suit I owned; one I had bought just a few months ago to attend an engagement party. It was a white skin-tight skirt and double breasted jacket that layered nicely in the front; a snug fit. It comfortably wrapped the curves of my body in its soft fabric. I liked this suit. I felt good in it, sexy even. My accompanying dark, strappy high heels were slightly too tight and constricted my toes, unnoticeable to others, but somewhat uncomfortable for me to walk in. They were my only option, so I slipped them on. I felt a bit like Cinderella going to the ball and my confidence stepped up a couple of notches.

I took one last long look in the mirror my eyes scanned for any imperfections. My lightly applied makeup perfectly matched my suit. I was happy with my reflection. I needed to at least look professional, even if I didn't feel it. I was particularly anxious, yet definitely excited. I started to visualise myself working in this resort. I wondered if it would be fun, or would it be mundane? I settled for fun. I pondered what I could do. Would I work in the bar, the nightclubs or the restaurants? Maybe, even the large conventions centre; I thought that would be exciting.

Off I went to meet the manager of this five star resort with hope and expectation in my heart. I knew this job would secure a future here on the Gold Coast for my daughter and me.

A proficient, well-dressed manager and a lovely, short-haired woman in her late thirties who wore a pink low-cut dress, greeted me. We spoke for over an hour. They both attempted to make me feel at ease, but my apprehension prevailed. Our conversation flowed smoothly and positively, however, I felt the volley and torrent of questions were more like an interrogation. I was lucky that I could think on my feet and expand stories quite easily. After the formalities were completed, the manger left me in the care of the small, warm and friendly supervisor, who I warmed to straight away.

She directed and physically escorted me to a beautiful, peaceful tropical barbecue area, where overhanging trees and customized, concrete garden paths surrounded me as I was shown the resort recreational area. I noticed personalized and well-tended flower gardens, full of colourful plants that overlooked two very large, crowded pools. In the centre of this beautiful sculptured garden, stood a large open, wooden, Balinese-style hut. A barbecue plate sizzled and erupted as red hot flames danced and licked aromatic steaks and sausages.

I noticed a tall, bearded man wearing a white loosely-fitting chef's outfit, as he calmly and conscientiously flipped small, searing, bleeding steaks. Another tall, dark-haired man in a pink, floral shirt and white, tight shorts leaned over the counter. They both cheerfully laughed at some insignificant, yet obviously humorous, topic, as I passed between them. My hungry eyes consumed the scene. My heart accelerated; the sound announced itself loud and clear in my ears. It's quickened pace forced intense heat to flood throughout my body, which flushed my cheeks as blood coloured my face. I couldn't take my eyes of the stunning, muscular being before me. Who was this guy?

Nothing mattered now; my focus completely engaged on the man in front of me. Everything else faded in the distance. My peripheral vision acknowledged, but no longer registered, the words that hovered. They were just letters that drifted like particles of spinning dust, illuminated by the rays of morning sunlight. Somewhere in the back of my mind I knew I should be listening, trying to grasp the concept of what I was being told. I knew these words had impact and meaning to my life, but this action eluded me.

The man in the chef's outfit noticed me first. His reaction was simple and primal. He looked intently at me, then he leant over the barbecue counter to speak directly into the ear of the dark-haired man. Both men scrutinized me, blatantly looking me up and down. As they surveyed the scene before them, whispered words passed between them. I was the focal point of discussion, positioned in their full view, the bright stage light focused directly on me and the audience stared.

A whistle pierced the still air, catching and absorbing my attention, a smile rose to my lips as I knew that it was intended for me. I couldn't be sure who actually issued the shrill note, but I secretly hoped that it would be the dark-haired man. It made my heart miss a beat, every cell tingled within me, fully awakened. They vibrated and pulsated in tune, fiery flames flickered and crept up my neck and around my cheeks turning them a blazing red. I allowed my long, lustrous, dark mane to partially conceal my face and cover some of my obvious awkwardness. My eyes dropped and firmly refocused on the heavy grey concrete beneath my feet. I was being lead out of the area by my disgusted escort. It was then that I realized that the woman was still talking. Her words became clearer, sharper and more coherent and she was offhandedly apologising for her employees' behaviour. I didn't mind. My interview was over. I looked back over my shoulder to have one last look, and then walked out the door.

My instructions were clear. I was to report back tomorrow for an induction, and commence work the same day. I was thrilled. I had done it! I didn't know how, but I had done something I didn't think was possible; I secured what I considered to be a decent job.

As I drove home, I contemplated the encouraging interruption of those two men and my heart fluttered slightly. I wondered if I would see them again. However, I knew that I needed to keep focused, simply because I needed this job to help secure a positive and productive life for myself and my daughter, and I could really not afford any form of distraction from that goal.

"I sit astride life like a bad rider on a horse. I only owe it to the horse's good nature that I am not thrown off at this very moment."

~Ludwig Wittgenstein

Chapter 24

Doubts

"Convert difficulties into opportunities, for difficulties are divine surgeries to make you better."
~author Unknown

My first day was full of laughter and fun. I was the new kid on the block; one who now wore a low-cut pink dress, and one everyone wanted a look at. Managers visited, staff dropped in, and curious customers questioned me and then gossiped about me openly. None of it could dampen my excitement. I was just thrilled to be working and to feel accepted by a really nice bunch of people.

I worked very closely with these two larger-than-life characters I had seen on that first day. The chef became my very best friend. He was charismatic, charming and funny, and the other one was an attractive, tall, quiet, dark-haired man who eventually stole my heart. We spent nearly every waking moment together; we worked, played and partied. I felt I had finally found somewhere where I could be accepted and felt wanted. I had found some sort of contentment. I would say I was even happy to some extent.

A few months passed, and I started to reflect on where my life was going. Had I made the right choice? This new life encompassed elements that terrified me. I doubted my ability to maintain any sort of positive relationship. My history was certainly very poor. Yes, I liked this guy, liked him a lot. But, was I going to be able to do something remotely constructive with him? Would he still like me if he really knew me? Could we have a real relationship, share a life together, one where I felt truly loved and accepted? Was that a possibility?

I liked my new 'straight' friends and I loved living on the Gold Coast. But was it going to be enough to prevent me from returning "home"? My daughter was settled and she had made some friends. Despite the secure new life that surrounded me, I still regularly had to fight the overwhelming desire to run away, which meant a return to the comfort and familiarity of my previous life.

Chapter 25

A gateway
"It has been my philosophy of life that difficulties vanish when faced boldly".
Isaac Asimov

A choice needed to be made and made soon. Could I trust myself enough not to sabotage this great thing I had, and could I trust him with my heart, or should I run like I had always done before? Guess what... I sabotaged my relationship. I actually pushed him away. My negative actions and dominating behaviours caused us to split up. I simply didn't feel that I was worthy enough to be with him. I had come from a relationship full of verbal and physical abuse and my self-esteem was misguided. I didn't know there was another way to live. Until I met this guy, my parent's relationship had also been volatile, so I thought that was normal in all relationships. But this guy was different in so many ways. He was kind, considerate, caring and gentle, and I didn't know how to react to that sort of behaviour.

During our time apart, I reconnected with a guy I had once known from Madang. We were good friends then, but had never really got together. I knew we had a spark between us, but we were from opposite ends of the spectrum. His dad and my dad played in a band together, and we spent a lot of nights hanging out, killing time. I had not seen him since I left in 1980, five years had passed, and a lot of things had changed since then. I was not the same person he knew in Madang. I had a troubled spirit and carried heavy burdens and internal dark passengers that regularly threatened to overwhelm me.

I don't know how he found me, but he did. I guess being a policeman helped. His phone call came, quite unexpectedly, asking to see me as he was now working in Brisbane. I was stunned that he had located me, yet, curious to see him again after all these years. So, we got together and spent the night trying to reconnect. We talked about everything, but the spark between us no longer lingered. It had died in Madang, along with my vitality and radiance, and we never saw or spoke to each other again.

Chapter 26

Crunch time

> *"These were people so hungry for love that they were accepting substitutes. There were embracing material things and expecting a sort of hug back. But it never works. You can't substitute material things for love or for gentleness or for tenderness or for a sense of comradeship.*
> ***Author unknown***

None of my life occurrences are unique. Many women experience similar situations and are faced with the same questions. How I approached my life, the choices I made and the sequence of events that followed these choices are what make this story unique. Previous experiences moulded my thoughts, influenced my feelings, unearthed my fears and gave birth to the outcomes that occurred.

I needed to make a choice. Did I trust something unknown to me, or something real and tangible that I knew? My choice was between returning to a familiar life, one that was well established, yet self-destructive and filled with hopelessness and limited possibilities. A life that offered nothing but despair and no visible lifelines that I could hold onto when the seas got rough. Or, I could stay and fight for a new life, with an unknown destiny, an unidentified objective with an unknown person, and me as the unexperienced driver.

I deliberated back and forth for quite some time. Should I return to what I knew or should I stay and see what happens? Decisions, decisions. I generally made decisions easily, especially when it was about something that I didn't really care about, but this one was a matter of the heart and didn't only affect me.

I finally made my decision. I would stay and see where this life took me. I would make no plans. I would allow the cards to fall where they may. So, I totally turned my back on my old ways. I rang my daughter's father and told him that I would not be returning, and that

I was severing all ties with him. I did not want, ask or expect support from him. I wanted to do this myself. Deep down I feared if I maintained any contact with him, that my resolve could falter, and I would return to that life of destruction. I was genuinely scared of the profound magnetism that that life had on me and how weak I still was. I could only hope that I would get stronger with time.

Was my decision aided by Divine intervention? I don't know, was it just my personality? I don't know. Was it a mother's instinct? I don't know. What I do know is that I chose a new life. I chose an unknown and untried trail, one that only I could discover.

Once the decision was made, I witnessed something powerful grow within me. I felt the bonds that held me to my old life crumble, and in its place stood a pillar with a deep, strong foundation. I felt a force drive me forward in confidence. I didn't understand it or know where it came from, I only knew that it gave me a strength and courage that I had never seen before in myself.

Seeds of doubt still lingered, but as time passed, I found it easier to suppress them, conquered by my new determination to succeed at this life I had chosen. I stripped off my old life, discarded it like my winter wardrobe in summer. A new person emerged, someone who I think was always there, but had lain dormant within me all these years.

Time stealthily moved forward. My summer wardrobe rapidly expanded, filled with fragrances of hope and optimism. Each new summer dress symbolized a positive experience, a conquered crisis, a triumph over a difficulty. As my outfits increased so did my self-esteem, which cultivated more confidence and optimism.
I found a new sense of purpose, a real goal. I wanted to live and be a good mother. My innocent babe, her hair black, the colour of a Spanish stallion, her immense beauty rivalling all others, needed a father who loved her, someone to provide guidance and stability to her previously unstable world, and, I needed to be emotionally fulfilled. So I forged a distinct path forward for both of us. I strode head first into a previously forbidden world. A world where love was mutually offered and accepted, and where distinct boundaries lay.

Optimism replaced negativism.

Chapter 27

A Fathers Pledge

"Lots of people want to ride with you in the limo, but what you want is someone who will take the bus with you when the limo breaks down."
~Oprah Winfrey

During the final year with the father of my child, I spent quite a lot of time rebuilding a relationship with my father. I realised that a loving family should find everything - well, most things - forgivable; it just takes a bit of time to move forward again. Our relationship was far from perfect but we had something tangible that I could believe in.

His final words to me continued to plague me. Questions rolled around in my mind. What did he mean by all of that "I am praying for you" stuff? Why did he say that to me? What did it all mean? I didn't understand this new man, this father of mine. He didn't even resemble the man I thought I knew as my father. The transformation was simply amazing. I wondered what had happened to him. He exhibited and displayed something that I longed for, internal peace and enlightenment. Joy now illuminated and radiated from his face, it replaced the veil of pain and the mask of suffering he once wore.

I didn't posses any of those features that I had observed in him; the changes so drastic they were hard to comprehend. I desperately desired what he had. Even though my life on the Gold Coast was better, I still had a very troubled heart, the storms in my life raged constantly and sleepless nights plagued me. My internal life was in complete disarray.

My dad's life was more like a light on a dark winter's day. Our last meeting replayed in my thoughts and lingered for many days. However, like all things, the memory eventually receded into the gloomy dark corners of my mind, overtaken by life's activities.

"Nothing is predestined: The obstacles of your past can become the gateways that lead to new beginnings."
Ralph Blum

Chapter 28

Learning to forgive

"In those times we yearn to have more in our lives, we should dwell on the things we already have. In doing so, we will often find that our lives are already full to overflowing."
- Jim Stovall

As my new life unfolded and my daughter settled into her positive environment, my internal demons started to surface. I started to doubt that the situation I was in would work out, and that it would eventually end up being meaningless, with unfulfilled expectations. The secrets I kept hidden continually shouted at me from within, reinforcing these doubts.

During these dark times, I sought solace in my father's promise: "I am praying for you." I didn't understand its meaning, but I knew that it was meant to uphold me somehow.

The relationship I shared with my parents over the last 24 years was quite unpredictable, explosive and unstable. The history that bound us was fraught with anguish, grief and hurt which caused us all to engage in a lot of conflict.

Conflict is a natural occurrence in life, one that is based on emotions and where energies interact, either positively or negatively. All of our conflicts were subjective, and were underpinned by individual perceptions, misinterpretations, poor communications and expressions, power, feelings and intentions.

As I look back on our family situation, I can see where we went wrong, and why we all became so estranged, but when you are living in a situation, it is hard to see a single tree in a thick forest.

I don't think any conflict should be a contest between parties. Rather, it should be used more as an opportunity to grow and learn. Unfortunately, this did not occur in my family. A battle of wills ensued, where neither side conceded, whereas, if we had learnt to communicate more effectively and listen to each other without judgment or criticism, we all might have changed the dynamics of the family as well as our thoughts and attitudes towards one another.

We may have learnt to be more accommodating, more flexible, more adaptable and communicate differently. Resolving conflict is rarely about who is right or wrong; it is about acknowledgment and appreciation of differences.

Reconnecting with my father taught me the real meaning of forgiveness. I came to realise that it is important to understand that we are all capable of making mistakes, and we do. We all suffer misfortunes in life whether they are due to our own hands or someone else's; it is simply a fact of life. Life is tough.

We sometimes act on misunderstood or partial information. We do and say stupid things that we later regret because of our emotions and insecurities, and in the process, the collateral damage is people, and usually, you hurt the person you love. There is a saying that goes, "hurt people hurt people". I know I did. I believe that it is up to us, as individuals to break that cycle, and that is what my dad did. He had the guts to come forth and identify and admit his part in the wreckage that had become my life.

When we choose to forgive, we change, and others change around us. Situations change, and that is certainly what happened to me and my parents. Learning to forgive them both was not easy, and it took a lot of ongoing work on my behalf. They had hurt me deeply. But as my father altered his attitude towards me, my behaviour also altered. I found I was more accepting of him and more forgiving, and deep down I realised I had missed his influence in my life and my daughters.

I also realised that blaming others for what is happening or has happened, doesn't get you anywhere. When you blame others, you point a finger at someone else, but three always point back at you. When I stopped blaming my parents for everything that was wrong in my life, I actually started to heal, and I was able to take some positive steps forward.

I lived with both guilt and blame which were equally destructive forces in my life. I hated being chained to the grudges and hurts of my childhood. I wanted to see the world through clear glass, not through the dirty glass that I currently viewed it through. To do this, I needed to forgive myself and stop the self-imposed punishment. My actions of the past were done and could never be undone, so I needed to find a way to live with my choices, and deal with the guilt that came with them.

Forgiving my mother took a lot more time and effort on my behalf, because she simply didn't demonstrate the remorse or sorrow that was obvious with my father. She reached out to me, but I was always reluctant to trust her intentions, searching for hidden agendas. However, in time, forgiveness filled my heart and I tentatively reengaged with them both. I dipped my toes in the water one at a time, taking things slowly, and what I found was that I could love them both from a distance.

I learnt that disasters aren't really disasters if you take them apart piece by piece, and that was what helped me along this path. Every time I thought or perceived something negative about our new found family relationship, I would pull it apart and scrutinise it piece by piece; this helped me to displace the negativity that terrorized me and the demons that whispered in my ear, speaking a pessimistic, unconstructive language.

> *"It is interesting to notice how some minds seem almost to create themselves, springing up under every disadvantage, and working their solitary but irresistible way through a thousand obstacles."*
>
> *- Washington Irving*

Chapter 29

Lightening and Fire connect

"Some people come into our lives and quickly go. Some stay for a while, leave footprints on our hearts, and we are never, ever the same."
~Flavia Weedn

I stood firm in my conviction and I would not give up. I had tried, and was still trying, to come to terms with the actions of the past, and I had now made a commitment to stay on the Gold Coast. I had purposefully shed the old fabric of my original life and replaced it with the allure and fascination of the Gold Coast's charm, as well as the new magnetism I felt for a dark-haired, well-built, broad-shouldered, quiet young man named John.

We were like lightening and fire, a mix of two negative reactions. He was like lightening, me like fire. Both of us brought baggage and heavy burdens into this union, but we forged forward anyway. Lightening is beautiful to watch, brilliant in stature and power, bright and fast. 70% of its powerful flashes occur internally and when the negative particles meet, they form a very jagged path splitting the sky in two. The man I loved was just like this. He had a brilliant mind, he was confident, had direction, goals and dreams. He was powerful in his own right, majestic even. Yet, he kept himself closed off from the world by cloudy barriers, like a safety net. He was slow to react, yet, just like lightening, 70% of his anger was internalized, and the dark clouds moved slowly overhead, and when released, it was definitely a force to be reckoned with.

At the time of our union, I was more like fire. I constantly manoeuvred and manipulated the world around me to achieve my goals and to feed my internal furnace; my temperament could be a blazing hot tornado amid the fiercest chaotic winds. My verbal, coiling flames could easily ignite any smouldering ash. I could also propel searing balls of heat to bring destruction to everything in its path. I am sometimes like an unstoppable monster which consumes at will, or a blazing firestorm that stealthily stalks and pursues and devours its prey. I have a fiery temperament which is covered by my intense passion. However, my personality sometimes lacks diplomacy. My tact can be severe, my thinking rigid and my perception destructive. Angry critical words can easily rumble forward off my tongue and set fire to any situation. I used to sit in judgment, whilst being intolerant and critical.

We were two very different people who came together to form a mighty mix. We were potential masters of destruction but also the manufacturers of creation. Lightening illuminates the sky, a constant reminder of the essence of heaven; it brings rain which is also the cleanser of life. From the remains and the ashes of fire, new growth emerges. An awakening occurs to rise up and forge a new path. New life brings changes and hope, which emphasizes expectation and anticipation.

"Wherever you are, be all there".

- Jim Elliot

Chapter 30

Unrestrained Addictions

"Character is like a tree and reputation like its shadow. The shadow is what we think of it; the tree is the real thing."
Abraham Lincoln

Even though I was satisfied with my present-day life and my current beau, I refused to stop drinking heavily. Working in the hospitality industry just fuelled and encouraged my addiction, as well as presenting me with daily opportunities to satisfy my inner cravings. John and I worked regular shift work and at times we were required to work double shifts. We had a pact: whoever finished first would wait at the bar for the other to finish, with the aim of dancing and drinking the night away in a local Surfer's Paradise bar. Cheap staff drinks were offered to all staff at our establishment, and we frequently overindulged ourselves as we debriefed after a long day.

One of those drinking sessions, assisted by over-exuberant work comrades, resulted in my incarceration. Living only a few blocks from my workplace, I left my workmates and drove erratically home which included driving a short distance up the Gold Coast Highway the wrong way, and nudging a post box before parking. After I had fallen out of the car, I was greeted by a curious police officer, who received a mouthful of abuse about my rights to privacy, and that he should mind his own #$%^&#@ business.

My only real recollection of the whole event was sitting in the staff bar drinking Ouzo and talking to my friend, the chef. I had planned to wait for John as per our arrangement, however, as I waited, the bar staff enhanced my drinks with excessive amounts of Ouzo and I abandoned any reason or restraint. A few hours later, I knew I needed the familiarity of home, so I embarked on a treacherous journey, driving a lethal weapon.

John finished his shift and I was not there, so he was completely unaware of the events that transpired or my whereabouts.

The morning dawned, my eyes were blurry, unable to focus, and my hazy mind was unable to comprehend my surroundings. I found myself lying on a very hard surface, like the floor, but it was a concrete cot secured to the wall. I noticed I was in a small, windowless, open-plan, besser block room with bars across the only opening which faced a long brightly lit hallway. It was then that I realised I was in jail.

I slowly sat up and tried to recall the details of last night's antics, but they wouldn't come forward, drowned in a sea of alcohol and swept away with the tide. A young girl sat in a cell directly across from me, staring intently, assessing my movements. My legs were unsteady, shaky as I rose to meet the uniformed officer who offered me a piece of cold toast lathered in vegemite and a cup of luke warm tea. I accepted these hand-outs, but was unable to consume any of them. I was more interested in the freedom that awaited me at the end of the presented phone.

Before I could be released I had to pay $330.00, which was an outstanding fine I had been issued in Townsville. My only option was to ring John, inform him of my behaviour, and ask if he could raise the money. Our phone conversation was very short, one-sided and filled with suggestions and condemnation. A compromise was recommended and a deal struck between us. He was irritated, disappointed and frustrated with me all at the same time, but he came for me, paid my passage and released me from my incarceration.

A lesson was eagerly taught but this student was unwilling to learn. Embarrassment, remorse and guilt overrode all my other emotions, until we arrived home. All these emotions totally forgotten, replaced by the silent call of my inner being, an appeal from the 'hair of the dog.' I was being summoned to ease my self-inflicted pain and suffering, a request I was unable to forgo.
I faced four charges as I left the police station, and a couple of days later, I was in court, ready for my sentence.

The court room resembled a large auditorium, seats ranged up the walls like a university lecture theatre. The judge presided over the proceedings from a podium located at the front. Numerous offenders like me decorated the rising seats, all awaiting judgment.

My tough sentence was now imposed. The judge took my licence for nine months and ordered me to pay $975.00, both were a challenge and hard to bear. The loss of my licence, a very tough warning, stripped me of my independence and freedom. It was a lesson I only needed to learn once, and it was one I would never repeat. His sentence prevented me from being able to engage with my friends or participate fully in my life, it forced me to totally rely on John, which disempowered me and removed my autonomy. This situation irritated him just as much as it frustrated and displeased me, but it didn't change my drinking habits.

Shortly after this imposed sentence, we decided to move into a flat closer to our work, which meant that driving was no longer necessary for either of us.

"Success in the affairs of life often serves to hide one's abilities, whereas adversity frequently gives one an opportunity to discover them."

Horace

Chapter 31

Decision time
"Living involves tearing up one rough draft after another."
~Author Unknown

Two years into our relationship, we started to discuss marriage and children. I suppose a natural progression for a connection like ours. We loved each other. We shared a deep, profound companionship and had begun to create some lasting memories. However, our relationship was far from perfect. Communication problems regularly plagued us as both of us had suppressed hurts which were sometimes corrosive to the relationship.

My un-revealed history was a persistent dark horse in our relationship, and his critical nature brought major problems into our union. I was quite happy to maintain the status quo, changing the symmetry of our lives really concerned me, and my fear of marriage and the level of commitment it held frightened me. Previous visions of my parents' failed relationship saturated my beliefs and altered my overall philosophy about the stability of marriage. However, my inner feelings conflicted with these beliefs and turned my sceptical thinking around.

If I was to triumph over my fear of what marriage represented, I would need to expose my secret identity and uncover all my classified activities. I discerned I could not enter into this level of commitment when it held secrets.

The idea of unearthing my deeply buried, rotting past petrified me, but the truth needed to be revealed, if we were to have a future together. The prospect of resurrecting my old skeletons brought forth some apprehension and concern. I wondered how he would react. What would he think of me once he knew everything? Would he run for the hills? I might have, if I was about to hear all the sordid details I was about to divulge.

"In the book of life, the answers aren't in the back".

~Charlie Brown

Chapter 32

A risk worth taking

"You cannot discover the purpose of life by asking someone else - the only way you'll ever get the right answer is by asking yourself."
~Terri Guillemets

Brilliant light illuminated a new day. It warmed the morning as we prepared for a sizzling barbecue breakfast and a sun-drenched day on the beach. Our position purposefully chosen and secured, so we could keep an eye on Jade. I noticed she had chosen to wear her favourite pair of blue and white striped swimming pants to come to the beach, I had offered many times to buy her other brightly coloured swimmers, but she refused, wanting to live in these well-worn ones instead. I watched as she carried her bucket and spade and impulsively and eagerly ran towards the beckoning sand. She fell hastily to her knees, the red plastic spade hovered beside her, poised to enthusiastically build any creative sand structure she envisioned. All the while her blue eyes constantly sought our attention and approval.

I reviewed my surroundings. I sat evaluating the circumstances and revisiting my internal checklist ready for my disclosure. We appeared like any other young family out enjoying the day. John, an innocent, unsuspicious man stood beside a sizzling barbecue plate and turned sausages as his child laughed and happily played in her own magnificent daydream. Towering over them stood the majestic Gold Coast's famous Magic Mountain. The picture before me was delightful and peaceful. I wanted to remain here suspended like this forever.

But I knew I couldn't. So, I positioned myself nervously in front of him, his arms naturally reached out to embrace me. My internal radar searched for any unidentified movements, or gestures that could signal and alert me to any threats. I held his gaze, for a long moment. I wondered what sort of verdict would be pronounced today. Would he rule in my favour? Could he reason and offer leniency, or would he judge with prejudice and intolerance? I comprehended that today my life lay in the balance, any moment now he could tip the scales and I could sink to the ground.

My story needed to be told, for I had selected him as my mate. There was no other option. He had won the battle, my heart was the prize. Losing him now would leave a wound deeper than I dared to think about. An ache I would carry for the rest of my life.

His tender eyes searched mine, questioning and waiting. Silence hung between us. I couldn't postpone it any longer. Rapid burst of disjointed words exploded from my mouth. He listened intently, then studied me quietly for a long time.

I felt relieved. Finally I had offloaded my hidden secrets. They were all now fully exposed to the man I loved. I watched his expression change as he tried to rationalise the facts presented before him. I could see the injury and wounds that my words caused him, and I realised both our values and principles would be under intense scrutiny.

His grey eyes pierced every inch of me. A discharged bullet struck my heart as I waited for the words to fall, the words I knew would crush me. It would be over, there would be no absolution for me, I saw it in his face. I braced myself. My body was tense with apprehension, ready for the blow to come. But, it never did. He continued to slowly turn the sausages. Silently, he processed the information whilst I waited nervously.

I glanced at my daughter. I marvelled at her innocence, joy and happiness. I wished some of it would find its way into my life, now. I had laid myself bare to John, stripped off all the protective clothing of the past and now I stood nakedly before him, open and waiting for his response.

He finally spoke, his voice hoarse and thick with emotion. His words surprised me. He simply stated none of it really mattered. What truly mattered was that he loved me. I was shocked by his response. My confession was fully heard and totally understood. Both mercy and compassion were offered to me and I accepted them. He did, however, put a stipulation on our relationship, one that I had no problem abiding with. He forcefully stated, if I ever took hard drugs again, such as using heroin, our relationship would be over. I couldn't believe it was that easy. It made me question why I didn't come clean sooner. He had offered me a chance I never thought I would get. Euphoria and ecstasy replaced my previous fear and doubts.

An enormous wave of relief swept over me, its swell surged over every inch of my being, drenching me with infinite freedom. I felt completely liberated. Life was now limitless. I ran to him and wrapped my arms tightly around him, pulling him intimately towards me and nestling my head closely into his exposed chest. I looked up into his eyes and vowed never to partake of any substances like that ever again, for I loved him deeply.

We were married early in 1988, my daughter was five. A new expedition began to unfold for all of us. It was a road less travelled, a path completely unknown to me, with no footprints to guide me. This time I would have to leave my own marks in the sand, never looking back. For the past is just that, and should be left where it falls. My pardon had been issued. I had been released from my convictions and there was no benefit in revisiting any of it ever again.

The three of us confidently advanced forward, knowing we would share excitement, fear, enjoyment, pain, growth and lots of love.

> *"The love of a family is life's greatest blessing"*
> *"Other things may change us, but we start and end with family"*
>
> ***Anthony Brand***

Chapter 33

Trouble in paradise
"Nothing matters to the man who says nothing matters"
Lin Yutang

A tragedy occurred in 1988, shortly after our marriage. It was aAn event which pounded and weakened the foundations of our newly formed union. My father-in-law was diagnosed with cancer and subsequently died a slow and painful death. John sat at his side, day after day, witnessing the pain and suffering his father endured.

John's world crashed around him. The bricks and mortar holding his life together started to fracture as he was struck by overwhelming grief and sorrow, both of which consumed and filled his life. His tortured soul set alight and burnt all other feelings. I found there was little room left for my daughter and I in his now tightly coiled life. We were outcasts, left standing alone, separated from his world. We became independent bystanders, powerless to comfort him as we observed his internal eruptions.

For a long time, I watched and waited as John slowly clawed his way back to me. He finally was able to battle his demons and dislodge them from their previously dominant position in his life. He transferred his grief and depression into an obsession with exercise. He started to run, running for hours to try and rid himself of the negative, depressive feelings that continued to hover and lurk in the background.

John wanted and needed direction, a career. So he joined the Army and we were moved to Toowoomba. This move isolated me and I found myself raising my daughter alone on an army base, with no support system, no friends and no job prospects. John's new position, as well as adapting to the Army culture, was stressful for all of us. His long hours, coupled with frequent trips away, resulted in him becoming more introverted, distracted and withdrawn from the family unit.

Army life prevented us from maintaining or rebuilding our

relationship, which had been seriously damaged after the death of his father. I craved company, so I started to create a social life 'outside' of the army culture. I secured a job which enabled me to meet new people and regain some independence. My newly created life didn't include John, as he was away more than he was home. I fostered meaningful relationships with others outside of our marriage which isolated and divided our family further and my marriage really started to suffer.

When John was home, communication between us was quite limited. We were two people who shared a house, with no common goals and no common purpose. I wondered what had happened to us. But I soon realised, I was living a life that resembled my parent's relationship. It was one I had vowed not to copy when I first entered into this marriage. I guess the frequent separations, our fragmented goals and shattered dreams, as well as our apathetic responses, resulted in both of us building two separate lives and contributed to the loss of what we once both cherished.

John began to drink heavily. He slipped into the army 'boozing' culture with ease. It reminded me of the Madang culture where my parents lost track of everything, and John was not interested in any of my opposition to his behaviour.

My life had begun to change. I no longer felt the same desire to drink, socialise and party like before. Watching John suffer during his time of grief made me realise there was more to life than one more party. I started studying at TAFE and attended evening classes to get a certificate in exercise physiology. These lessons enlightened me about the importance of maintaining a healthy lifestyle and the benefits it could bring. All of this was in direct opposition to what my partner was doing and what I had previously done.

A couple of months into this course, I decided to become a vegetarian and adopt a real healthy lifestyle. This was a life John was not remotely interested in. He knuckled down and so did I. There appeared to be no compromise for us on the horizon. He continued on his path and I continued on mine.

I became increasingly unhappy. I tried to refocus all this unhappiness into work, which transformed me into a workaholic. I traded my addiction to drugs and alcohol for the achievement of goals. I had become a fitness instructor who taught up to thirty classes a week, worked weekends at a local golf club and managed a catering business. I would coerce, push and direct myself to achieve, achieve and achieve. This just caused me to become physically and mentally exhausted.

During those first couple of years when John was in the army, we spent less and less time together, and a distinct wedge grew between us. We spent more and more time with others pursuing our own interests. Separating would have been an easy option for us both at this point, as there was no glue that held us together anymore. Our marriage was basically over in principle, just not formalised on paper. We did actually part for a brief period, but for some reason we didn't separate permanently. My theory was a bond still held us together, even though it wasn't apparent, its substance unknown, yet, it reunited us and reignited the fire and passion in both of us.

"Treat people as if they were what they ought to be and you help them to become what they are capable of being."

Johann Wolfgang von Goethe

Chapter 34

Another path is offered yet unaccepted
"Life asks of every individual to make a contribution and it's up to that individual to discover what it should be"
Viktor Frankl

At the same time as we were reuniting, a young family moved in next door to us. I found myself drawn to the young girl's charismatic personality. Her name was Sue, and she was younger than me with two children and pregnant with another. There was something very different about her. She stood out from the rest of the army wives. Serenity, happiness and peace surrounded her, yet her living conditions were exactly like mine. Our husbands did the same job, our houses were cramped and confining and both of us were parents.

What did she have that I didn't? What I noticed was, she saw the positives in everything, even when life was turbulent and lonely. Her passion and commitment to her marriage and children was unmistakable and remarkable.

We talked a lot. At first just over the fence, then over a quick coffee, and later I found I spent a big part of my day with her. She really interested me. We shared our experience and discussed almost anything. However, I still withheld the restricted, deeply hidden secrets of my past. Those darker topics I would not share with anyone, they were in a bottomless cavern, unattainable and out of sight. The difficulties we faced were the main topics of discussion.

During one of these sessions, I came to realise just how much patience and empathy she had for others - something I had never considered in my self-centred existence. I wondered why. I cared about people in my own way. I just couldn't display it the way she did. What was so different about me? Why wasn't I like her? I found myself constantly comparing myself to others, especially those that appeared to be really happy. I wasn't entirely unhappy with my life, so, why wasn't I as happy and contented as so many others around me? I should have been, John and I were getting on really well but…

Sue opened up to me one day, and explained she was a Christian. I questioned what that meant. She described how she chose to live her life with hope instead of in fear. A concept I had never considered before. She went on and rationalized that faith was the conviction that things which are anticipated, but currently unseen, will come to pass. I didn't understand her words. They might as well have been double Dutch, for I could not grasp their meaning. I needed time to digest her statement. I mulled it over for weeks trying to find its true meaning, before I came back and debated this philosophy with her.

My analysis came back to the belief that people always have a choice in life, they either choose a life full of fear or a life of hope. They either step out in faith or they stay hidden, never changing or growing. It is just as hard to choose a life full of fear, as it is to choose a life full of faith. She said that faith teaches that you are not the centre of the universe, but something bigger directs events around you, whilst it layers you in a blanket of love. Wow! This blew me away, and once again I went away challenged and contemplative.

One day, unexpectedly, she quite matter-of-factly informed me that she was praying for John and me to have another child. Her next statement took me by surprise, as it was completely outrageous, but somewhere in the back of my mind it sparked a desire and hope. She told me I would soon fall pregnant and have a son. I thought this was laughable since we had been trying on and off for years. Incredibly, a couple of weeks later her premonition about my pregnancy came true!

This made me question everything I thought I knew and believed in. I believed in a higher power, but a God like she knew, that was something totally different. When my child was born and I saw it was a boy, her words stirred within me. They reawakened a belief system that I heard about once before from my father. I began to think that maybe, just maybe, there was something to this God thing.

How could I not believe? Something had occurred, because a baby boy, a promised child, lay in my arms. Gazing into his beautiful face I started to understand I truly was not the centre of this universe. The world did not revolve around me or my little unit, but there was something much, much bigger in the world than I had ever imagined. I reflected often on our talks and the seeds she planted in my life. However, her seeds were sown on barren ground, unable to produce deep roots, and the plants they produced were unproductive and fruitless, and like my father's words before them, they faded into the background of my life.

This was a turning point in my life. A hand had been offered to me, but my arrogance and pride overruled any sound judgment. They prevented me from pursuing something I desperately needed: guidance and wisdom.

Sue enjoyed and possessed a life that was full of wisdom. I witnessed it daily as I observed the way she lived and interacted with others. She had shown me a life full of promise, hope and grace. However, when our lives parted, the cares of the world triggered a case of amnesia, and I forgot everything I had previously seen. As a result of my ignorance and lack of desire to change, I found myself in a continual cycle of destruction. My life was like a yo-yo. I was up one moment and down the next. I could find no even rhythm to help me. Over the next ten years, this would not change. Our location would, but our lives wouldn't, we were trapped in this cycle.

My fiery, domineering nature continued. I was slapped in the face a few times, beaten by life situations and taught some tough lessons, but none of them were tough enough for me to stop and start dealing with my internal baggage, or stop and focus on what really mattered in life. I was just like the Eveready bunny. I kept on the same path, at the same speed going nowhere, until one day, the cold surface of a sledge hammer struck me. It broke my spirit and forced me to stop and listen.

"Our most basic instinct is not for survival but for family. Most of us would give our own life for the survival of a family member, yet we lead our daily life too often as if we take our family for granted."

~Paul Pearshall

Chapter 35

Self obsession

"Acknowledge that you failed, draw your lessons from it, and use it to your advantage to make sure it never happens again."
- Michael Johnson

I spent my 30's and early 40's working, working and working. I also studied as I tried to find myself. Work became my primary focus and I lost sight of everything else in my life. I thought all my achievements would be enough retribution for all the wrongful deeds I had committed. I believed I could buy my way out of all my sins by achieving greater and greater things. I thought people would notice and I would feel fulfilled, but I found the more accolades that hung on my wall, the emptier I felt. I desperately sought validation and acceptance. I wrongfully believed my deeds would bring integrity into my life, but they didn't.

Throughout these two decades, I became more and more autonomous, self-sufficient and independent, isolating myself and living my own life. I simply and easily pushed my family away. I lived my life selfishly and lost sight of what truly mattered. These years were surrounded by turmoil and hardship simply because I failed to listen to the internal voices telling me to change. I was trapped in the currents of my negativity and destructive patterns, unable to forgive myself and move on. As I stood at the top of my lonely mountain, I glimpsed the promises of restoration, but failed to fully trust that they would help me. I refused to explore the possibilities of a new way of life, trapped in my defiant, self-defeating frame of mind. I simply refused to venture into or believe in things unseen or unproven.

"Nobody has ever before asked the nuclear family to live all by itself in a box the way we do. With no relatives, no support, we've put it in an impossible situation."

~Margaret Mead

Chapter 36

Alpha and Omega
"Beginnings are often scary, endings are often sad, but it's the middle that counts. You should remember that when you find yourself at the beginning."
Steven Rogers

In my early 40's, after much self-reflection and a failed business, I substituted my health and fitness career of fifteen years for a slower paced position which offered more time and a stable income for the growing financial demands of our family. I did, however, maintain a small personal training business which operated around my new employment. I had a contract with the state government working in the prison and correctional system. The pay was mediocre, but government work offered me some job security. The decision to change careers was to radically transform not only my life, but, the life of my immediate and extended family.

I found working for Corrections to be overly controlled, monitored and highly structured. It was a system that didn't allow for resourcefulness, innovation or divergence from the rules, regulations, procedures or time schedules. It confined not only the prisoners, but the staff as well. Emotionally and physically, I struggled under the weight of this oppression. My sanctity became more intensive study and I completed the Correctional Diploma in record time.

As Correctional Officers, we had many daily mundane duties, such as sitting for long periods of time as we babysat prisoners, who interacted in the playground of incarceration away from society. We wrote reports, filled in logbooks and drank lots of coffee. Sound exciting? This was not Hollywood. Tom Selleck's portrayal of the prison system in "An Innocent Man" was not what I saw. Communal showers did not exist and they were not hunting grounds, nor were there any George Clooney/ Brad Pitt type masterminds plotting a series of Casino heists. In reality I found it boring, completely unstimulating and un-motivating. However, there were days when I felt fully alive. Adrenalin coursed through every inch of my body as events unfolded. Clandestine activities occurred such as illicit drug trafficking, acts of retribution, assaults and power struggles, as well as taboo relationships. These acts facilitated regular cell searches, targeted urine testing, drug busts and sometimes officer assaults. Drug paraphernalia and tattoo equipment posed the biggest threat to staff in our daily routines through the risk of blood-borne virus exposure.

The impact of the sledgehammer's blow hit me with full force one evening whilst working in this new profession. My whole life would be turned upside down, radically changed.
It was the last shift of my roster. I contemplated my upcoming three days off as I walked up the wire-encased walkway. I passed through the large, centrally controlled, heavy steel gates, said hello to my fellow officers and casually strolled to my designated work area. The morning briefing began with a review of the previous day's activities and the days expected outcomes, including a cell search schedule.

The supervisor informed us, we were not to release any prisoners from their cells until we had thoroughly searched each unit and each cell. We were specifically instructed to look for drugs and any drug paraphernalia. Dread filled me. I hated these sorts of days, but they had become a regular occurrence. These events always irritated and frustrated the prisoners and some became so infuriated with their situation they became aggressive and abusive. They felt disempowered as we sorted through all of their personal effects and removed any items of interest. It was one of those times when we were required to strip all bedding, as well as urine-test targeted prisoners. I acknowledged that this would be a very long day, most likely with lots of paperwork. What made it worse was that the riot squad, including the service dogs, would be involved, so it had the potential to turn horribly wrong...... violent. I knew an incident would most likely occur. I only hoped it wouldn't be in my unit, as I despised all the paperwork involved.

We were partnered up. Six officers, including myself, searched a block of units. We found nothing significant except excess clothing and other items not belonging to the specified prisoner. Those items were removed and 'bagged and tagged' for return to the stores area. My partner wanted a coffee, so I decided to walk the confiscated items up to the supervisor's office for further processing.

I picked up the heavy, cumbersome white sheet containing allcontaining all the confiscated items and slowly walked up the walkway. As I moved towards the gate I felt an intense burst of pain, like a wasp sting on the outside of my thigh. I looked down to see a sharp object sticking out of the sheet, it was not a needle, but it was an implement used for prisoner tattooing. It had obviously not been secured properly. The contents of the package must have dislodged as I moved up the walk way, making it possible for the sharp implement to pierce through my clothing and jab my thigh.

The gates of the normally secured area were ajar, and I walked easily into the control room. Two officers sat managing the touch screen computers, electronically opening cell doors and recording events within the six units. The supervisor sat behind them overseeing all actions. I found it impossible to look at any of them as my mind raced with the dire possibilities of what had happened on the walkway. Luckily everyone was far too busy to notice me.

I dropped the bundle of goods into the adjacent supervisor's office and quickly went into the toilet to assess my injury. I removed my starched uniform pants to look at my thigh. I noticed a raised, swollen patch and some coagulated blood concealing a small open wound. I knew then, with absolute certainty, the sharp instrument in the bundle had caused the injury. Possibilities raced through my mind. The potential exposure to an infection dominated my thoughts.

I sat in stunned silence. Disbelief and apprehension swept over every part of me. The small cubicle closed in around me, crushing me. The cold steel toilet seat offered a small comfort to my growing concern.

I thought of many things during those first few seconds. My family, my life, my health, my friends, all of them flashed before my eyes. I knew a lot of prisoners were infected with Hepatitis C (HCV) and HIV. Up to 60% of them were infected with one of them. But, what were the risks to me? I didn't know. HIV screamed its name at me. Oh my God. What would I do if I got HIV? I knew a lot more about HIV than the hepatitis's. I tried to think of anybody I knew who had come in contact with any of these diseases. I couldn't recall one name. I didn't know anyone. Images of the frightening 1980s Grim Reaper campaign, where unsuspecting people from all walks of life cowered on a bowling lane and waited for the Grim Reaper to bowl them over, completely shattered my resolve. I became frightened and upset.

I tried to pull myself together as I slowly emerged from the toilet. Panic threatened to take over my already unstable mind. I was unnerved and getting more flustered by the minute. Tremors crept up my body in slow moving waves. The supervisor looked up and noticed my condition and summoned me into his room. He saw how visibly shaken I was, and asked what had happened. The words describing what happened discharged from my mouth, like a rapidly firing weapon. He ordered me to go immediately to the medical centre for assessment.

The centre was in full lockdown, which meant movement to the lower part of the prison would be quicker and easier, as the concrete and wire-enclosed walkways would be silent and abandoned. I wandered alone and unaccompanied down the long, secluded passageways, through the huge steel gates and onto the medical centre. A friendly nurse greeted me at the door. I hardly recognised her as she ushered me into the waiting room. My mind was busy trying to recall what I had learnt about blood-borne viruses. What were they? How did you get them? My mind drew a blank. I couldn't recollect any information at all. I became very anxious and nervous. Fear was now the dominant emotion within me.

I knew Corrections had a negative culture when it came to Blood-Borne Viruses. Officers perceived a huge potential risk of infection by working in confined spaces and associating closely with infected prisoners. The subject was never openly discussed, but we all knew that prison rates of blood-borne viruses were higher than in the community. Both within the community and within my workplace there was a negative social stigma around these diseases. I was scared of how people would perceive me if I was to become infected. I felt that if I became infected, I would be shunned by not only my work mates and my family, but also the rest of society. How could I work and live amongst other people who would fear me, fear what I carried, fear what I could potentially give them. I feared it myself. What was I going to do if I picked up something? How could I let this happen to myself? I relived every step I had taken. I felt stupid, foolish for my actions, and I questioned if I could have done something differently?

The nurse broke through my reflection and asked me what I needed. Her eyes scanned my face as she assessed my behaviour. I retold my story in detail. She led me into a large, well-lit room, with a centralized, sturdy examination bed. Floor to ceiling shelves decorated the walls and were full of surgical implements and dressings. I lay on the table, removed my stiff uniform pants and allowed her access to my injury.

She swabbed and cleaned my wound as I waited for her verdict. She smiled and then hesitantly touched my shoulder for the briefest of moments, her soft contact reassured me. Her words were sympathetic as she explained I definitely had a deep puncture wound to the thigh. She instructed me to go to my local GP and get tested for Blood-Borne Viruses' (BBV'S). She also went on to briefly explain that the chance of contracting a blood borne virus was minimal, and I shouldn't be overly concerned.

She spoke sketchily about HCV/HIV but my mind was unable to comprehend any more information. It was too busy visualising disastrous scenarios. I needed to get out of there. I wanted time to be alone to think. She repeated her statement "the risks of contracting something, anything at all, are minimal." However, my apprehension grew, regardless of these words.

She presented me with an option to go home, or stay and finish the day. My mind processed through a quick check list; home alone to wallow waiting for a doctor's appointment, or pass the day and return to work. I took the second option, and chose to keep myself busy. I knew I had three days off tomorrow, so I could deal with the situation then. Right now, I needed distractions, and lots of them.

I completed all the formalities, the necessary paperwork, and left to return to my work unit. The slow walk offered me private time to think, clear my head and make distinct future plans which would start tomorrow by getting the necessary test done.

I arrived at the unit to find my morning prediction correct. Rowdy, boisterous prisoners flaunted troublemaking activities in front of annoyed officers. A rebellious group within a neighbouring unit attentively stalked an unsuspecting victim and assaulted him, causing mayhem within the unit. Alert officers signalled for assistance, and I found myself caught up in responding to the needs of others and forgetting about my personal plight, just like I had hoped for.

"Therefore do not worry about tomorrow, for tomorrow will worry about its own things. Sufficient for the day is its own trouble."

Matthew 6:34 NKJV

Chapter 37

Homeward Bound
"Love is a miracle, a vision to see"
Sheila Walsh

The day finally finished. Twelve hours had been successfully completed. The commander's voice announced that all was secured, and offered us our own freedom from our labour. Officers quickly scurried to their vehicles, eager to return home, me included. My homeward journey was overtaken by my thoughts and reflections of the chaotic day's events, my own personal incident temporarily forgotten. But as I turned my car into the long driveway leading up to my house, the memories and feelings flooded back. The recollections overwhelmed me. I sat for a few minutes in the car as I contemplated what I would say to John. I regrouped and restated words in my head, to try and create a coherent sentence of explanation.

Out of the corner of my eye, I saw movement. John had inquisitively come out of the house to see what was taking me so long, why I remained sitting in the car. He opened the door, his eyes searched for an explanation. A gush of rehearsed words cascaded from my lips formulating themselves into understandable phrases. My bomb was dropped on an unsuspecting man.

John had a way of doing what I least expect and this situation was no exception. He reached into the cold vehicle and purposefully grabbed my hand. His large warm hand engulfed mine, pulling and guiding me out of the car. He drew my trembling body to his steadfast mass, wrapped his muscular arms around me, and slowly leant forward to kiss my tear stained face and expectant lips. His solid, unwavering presence, as well as his words, comforted me. I felt safe in his arms; he was a soft warm blanket on a cold winter's night. Together, we would meet this head on, together, we could conquer whatever was dealt us, and together, hand in hand, we walked into the house, united against a common enemy.

Over a light dinner and a glass of red wine, we discussed the whole distasteful scenario. We pulled it apart, assessed every detail and analysed it. Here with my dependable husband, in the safety of my home, I didn't feel troubled or apprehensive. Both of us believed the chances of me contracting anything were very small, impossible even, and both of us dismissed the whole scenario.

I made the appointment and saw my local GP. He explained that it was highly unlikely I had picked up anything, but we still needed to go through the testing process anyway. I gathered the paperwork and drove to the pathology lab and had my blood taken, testing for HIV, HBV, HCV as well as syphilis.

My GP wasn't overly concerned, and this alleviated my alarm. Before I knew it, my three days off were over and I found myself back at work, experiencing another monotonous, yet busy, day. The day drew to an end and I was eager to obtain my freedom. I found myself leading the mass exodus of officers as they converged on the front gate. I reached my car and sat peacefully, watching car after car hurriedly dart towards the exit. I turned the radio on, Billy Idol belted out one of my favourite tunes. I turned it up, words blasted my ears and I sang tunelessly along with every word. The song ended, I started the car and set my sights on John at home.

As I drove home, I allowed peaceful thoughts to cleanse me of my day in prison. I arrived home and walked into the house, releasing myself from the constrictive uniform I was required to wear. As I walked down the slated narrow hallway and into the spare room, I yelled my usual welcoming greeting to John. I casually placed my work bag on the spare bed and hung the uniform on the hangers ready for the next day's use. I felt John's presence behind me.

Smiling, I turned. In front of me stood an anxious, distressed person, not the man I expected to see as I returned home. He stepped forward and grabbed me by the shoulders. His green-grey eyes penetrated and pierced me with a silent, deep stare. He cleared his throat and I knew he had something important to tell me. His voice was soft, kind, but direct. He said, "the doctor has left numerous phone messages for you to urgently contact him." I quietly listened to his words, knowing they were of significant importance, and tried to find and comprehend their hidden meaning, but couldn't. I silently wondered why the doctor would want to speak to me.

John had saved all the messages for me. I hastily brushed past him, lightly touching his shoulder as I ran to the kitchen where the cordless phone lay strewn haphazardly on the counter. I grabbed it. It seemed heavier than normal, burdened with a torrent of news it would soon pour into my ear. It burnt and sizzled in my hand as I dialled the numbers. Why this urgency to call him? What had happened? Was this about my test results? It couldn't be! I had chosen to put it, the incident, away from my mind, discarding it like it didn't really matter. But it was obviously now going to come back and haunt me.

Could I have picked something up from the incident at work? No, surely not. I couldn't have. Everyone I had spoken to about the incident reassured me that it was nearly impossible. I guess the word 'nearly' is just that, nearly, meaning that there was still a small risk. I didn't think of it in that context, I presumed I would be fine and in the impossible category, not the nearly impossible category.

My head spun as it tried to process all the thoughts. Too many scenarios rippled like thunder across the contours of my mind. Apprehension quickly swept over me. Hot rushes of adrenalin ascended and surged throughout my body. My skin became coated in a light lather of sweat and my muscles tensed ready to flee. I had HIV. It was the only possible answer for the doctor's calls. This thought terrified me. What did this mean to me and my family?

"Every second you dwell on the past you steal from your future. Every minute you spend focusing on your problems you take away from finding your solutions".

Robin Sharma, Who Will Cry When You Die?

Chapter 38

A mirror shatters

"Sometimes in tragedy we find our life's purpose - the eye sheds a tear to find its focus."
~Robert Brault,

I gathered my strength and stood in the kitchen to listen to the three saved messages. The doctor's tone was obviously disturbed, troubled, flustered even, behaviour completely unlike him. I looked up at the clock to assess the time. It was probably far too late to call the surgery, but I knew I would try anyway, I had nothing to lose.

Doubtful, but I dialled the number anyway. I waited as the phone rang an unrelenting tone in my ear. To my amazement, the phone was answered. A light, cheerful voice responded to the call and enquired about my needs. I explained who I was and that my call was in response to three requests from the doctor to call as soon as possible. She listened intently for a few moments then placed my call on hold for what felt like an eternity. Out of the blue, my call was suddenly redirected to the doctor's office. I was startled to hear the voice of my regular doctor. I never imagined he would still be at work at 7pm. I thought another doctor would have taken my call and offered an explanation as to why I was required to call, but here I was talking with the man himself. Shock and disbelief flavoured my tone as I spoke with him.

He explained he had something important to tell me, but it had to be done in person, and I was to come down to the surgery first thing in the morning. I told him I couldn't wait that long, I had to go to work in the morning so would not be able to come down until after this round at work. I told him I needed to know NOW. I was already extremely stressed, emotional and tormenting myself, thinking the worst. Sleep would be virtually impossible, as I couldn't go to bed with an unknown burden like this hanging over my head. I continued to coerce and manipulate him, overcoming all his objections with my quick rationalisations. Eventually, he broke under the weight of my convictions.

I used terms like, "I've got HIV haven't I? How long have I got?" I bombarded and assaulted him with these questions until I heard his agreeable and friendly Egyptian tone bite into my barrage. He said to me, "you really need to come and see me tomorrow."
I answered him, "what is going on? Do I or don't I have HIV?" His reply brought me to my knees. He said, "NO you don't have HIV. Your Hepatitis C (HCV) test came back positive, but this doesn't mean you have HCV, we will need to do the test again to make sure."

I could no longer speak. My words floated in the air around me, caught in the flakes of dust. My body felt like it was temporarily frozen in time. I was a statue. Six hundred and fifty words soared and glided effortlessly through my mind. Synapses fired simultaneously, as they all tried to reason and process this very raw, but very important, data. Accusatory statements started to form, and an internal critical and judgmental dialogue commenced, "you deserve this because of what you did all those years ago. See........ you will never amount to anything."

I vaguely heard the doctor say he wanted to make sure the diagnosis was correct by ordering another test. He wanted to be sure. Sure of what? What did that all mean? I wanted to be sure this wasn't all a mistake as well.

I slid down the wooden cupboards, my legs folded beneath me unable to hold the cumbersome weight placed upon them. I struck the icy, unyielding, slate floor. My hand still held the phone in a tight grip. My vision blurred as a steamy fog threatened to overcome me; air trapped deep in my lungs was unable to escape and caused my breathing to stop temporarily.

I finally found my voice and told him I would visit him in the morning and then our connection was lost. I was left speechless, dumbfounded as I sat on the floor. I had become a lump of un-sculpted clay, waiting for the moulding process to begin, I needed John to come and reshape my life to the way it was before this phone call. Was this really happening? Did I hear him correctly? Did he just say I had Hepatitis C? What the hell was that anyway?

I heaved my massively heavy burden off the floor. I stood and placed the phone, the jagged dagger that had pierced my world, back into its cradle. The house in which I stood became a super nova, a gaping black hole that threatened to suck me into it. I tried to navigate my way through the space continuum of my brain, but was unsuccessful as a mental haze had descended, blanketing logic and common sense with a vague emptiness. Sporadic questions fired into the deafening silence. Why? What was this all about? What was I going to do? What did this all mean? Was I going to die? What about my family? Why me? I repeatedly asked myself. No answers arose from the darkness.

What would happen to me now? My world, the mirror I was so accustomed to, the appearance I had spent so much time creating, shattered all around me. It took my dreams, my desires and my goals with it and threw them in pieces on the floor. My familiar image, the reflection I looked at daily, gone forever, smashed beyond repair. The tiny bits of ruined glass represented a time to create a new destiny, a new life that must arise from the ruins.

From the depths of my mind, I recalled Pamela Anderson had HCV. By all accounts, from what I had read in the tabloids, she was healthy and she didn't appear to really look after herself, she partied hard and drunk excessively. Whereas I exercised daily, ate well and didn't drink much. So, just maybe, things would be okay for me.

My recollection about HCV was very limited. I knew it was a serious disease, but I wondered about mortality. Did it kill people? Would it kill me? Would I become ill and die? Would I suffer? How painful would it be, or become? My kids, how was I going to tell them? What about all the things I wanted to do with my life, the places I wanted to visit, the people I would never meet, my career, my husband? The unstoppable questions just kept coming, like cannon balls striking my embattled ship. My vessel was damaged and wounded, but it refused to sink.

John intuitively realised I was ready to self-implode. He stepped from his vantage point and demanded my full attention by standing dutifully and dependably beside me. Slowly, he reached out and affectionately took my hand in his, turned it over, toyed with my fingers and gently stroked my palm. A blanket of silence covered us. No words could be spoken. He lingered, patiently caressing my hand waiting for the first words to come. Speech didn't come easily. My throat was painfully constricted with grief and my voice was ragged with anguish.

Humbly, my eyes full of shame, I turned and glanced up into his receptive face. His eyes revealed only his concern and love for me, not the expected condemnation I thought I would see. My mouth opened ready to speak, but instead, a waterfall of tears tumbled down my cheeks. Emotional barriers strangled every word as they slowly trickled from me. Jumbled sounds, undecipherable to me, but clear to him, flowed into pools of comprehensible statements. We both clearly understood I had HCV, although neither of us quite knew what this actually meant.

He embraced me, held me close, tight in his arms, and I could hear the steady rhythm of his heart, which comforted me. Together, we had weathered many storms, crossed many sandy deserts, and this would be no different. We had each other and the strength and courage to fight on. That was all that mattered. We believed taht together we would triumph over this adversity. This was merely a hiccup in our lives and we would deal with it like all the others we had faced before it.

The life I thought I knew was destroyed in an instant. The fiery flames that lingered constantly in the background of my life shot forward and devoured everything familiar to me, leaving only a single root to create a new destiny, a new life, which only I could bring forth from the ashes.

> *"I have always found that mercy bears richer fruits than strict justice."*
>
> *- Abraham Lincoln*

Chapter 39

Times of trial
"God pours life into death and death into life without a drop being spilled."
~*Author Unknown*

The hammer had struck a major blow to both our lives. We found ourselves in unchartered waters, new territory for us as a couple and our marriage. I knew this challenge would challenge both of us. I was unsure if our relationship, or even I, could weather these turbulent seas. If we did manage to conquer this milestone together, I knew we would be changed in undefined and unbelievable ways. I would never be the same. I also wondered how it would affect John and the rest of the family. My life had become a scene in a horrible, frightening nightmare; one where the main character, me, was tormented by shattered dreams and visions of doom and horror.

I was retested and returned a positive result. I must say, I expected this result, so it did not shock me. I was referred to a liver specialist, a gastroenterologist, specialising in HCV. The appointment was made for the next available date, which was four months away. I couldn't believe I would have to wait that long, but I did. No information was provided; no brochures or any other resources were readily available for me, simply because the GP had none. I found this whole initial process terrifying. I was not only scared, but shocked and traumatized by the whole event, and waiting four months to get any answers only added more stress. I had limited knowledge about the disease I carried and I needed to understand what would happen, today, not in four months.

I found myself in an impossible situation; one which disempowered me. My compassionate GP was unable to help me, as it wasn't his area of expertise, so I was left alone to fend for myself. I felt like I was living on another planet, a land that time and people forgot. I was so lost, so vulnerable, so alone and unable to share my situation with anyone. I didn't know where or whom I could get information from. Who could I talk to? I was too scared to talk to anyone, as I did not want them to judge me. I knew the social stigma HCV held. I worked in a culture of intolerance and judgment, so who could I turn to? I couldn't think of one person, not one. What was I going to do? Over the space of a week, my life had radically changed. A week ago I was happy, content, now I felt defenceless and weakened. I wanted to run and never look back, just like Forrest Gump did. Run from this disease, run from my life. I wished I could go back in time to a week prior, further even, back to when this all began, so I could change it. But none of that was a possibility. I had to play the cards I was dealt. I hoped I would have a winning hand sometime.

"You must rise above present discouragement and keep driving steadily and cheerfully forward, as all great persons have had to do."

Dorothea Kopplin, Something to Live By.

Chapter 40

Fears arise

"Here is the test to find whether your mission on earth is finished. If you're alive, it isn't".
~Richard Bach

The shoots of my past started to rise from the decaying ground. Condemnation surrounded me, and failure and hopelessness lived within me. They threatened the forgiveness John had given me all those years ago. I believed I was a failure as a wife, a woman and a mother. I knew I had brought disgrace, dishonour and scandal to John and our family. I questioned, how could I live with him when I thought he despised me as much as I despised myself?

Internally, the darkness matured. It obscured, suppressed and restrained the old me, and gave birth to a blemished, defective me. It rose like a monster, overpowering my whole being, stealing my mind, destroying my body and suppressing my soul. Feelings of conviction, contamination, dirtiness and despair sprouted. I just wanted to take a large, hard, bristled brush, and scrub myself clean, both inside and out, but I knew it would make no difference. These feelings flourished and overwhelmed me. I was the one who was usually in control, decisive, independent, and now I didn't know what to do or how to act.

I had to maintain the appearance of a normal life to the outside world, even though this diagnosis had turned my world into chaos. My life was a mess and I knew it. However, I still needed to go to work and function, which meant deceiving the people around me. This meant I had to become the old, familiar chameleon again. I put on a tightly controlled mask, and no one was alerted to the truth of what we were going through.

However, I struggled to maintain this front with people who really knew me, people I had grown fond of over the years and built a relationship with, such as my personal training clients. They could see I wrestled with something personal. In front of them, it became increasingly harder to pretend that everything was okay. So, I made the decision to finalise my business and told them all to go. This was a very hard thing for me to do, as some of them had become close friends. I wrestled with this decision, but ultimately, I knew I could not maintain the facade with them. I simply wasn't ready to reveal the truth about my past and my diagnosis, as I was still trying to come to terms with it myself.

I realised I could no longer effectively create programs for clients that needed constant positive reinforcement. If anyone was going to recognize a problem it would be these people. I feared their rejection and I wasn't ready for any questions. I didn't want our friendship to change, and I perceived it would if they knew everything. So, I chose to isolate myself and withdraw from them.

I despised myself for lying to them about the reason for closing the business, but I was unable to be truthful.

Days flowed into weeks. It became easier to mask my true feelings by portraying optimism, but internally, I was slowly eroding away. My self-confidence took a beating by my diagnosis. I didn't believe anyone would understand, or accept me, or what I was experiencing. Therefore, I found it easier to internalize my thoughts and my true feelings, and not reveal anything to anyone, not even my own children or other family members.

I became quite withdrawn, keeping everything locked away in a personally created bank vault, one only I could access. I pretended I was fine. My major fear was rejection. I knew I was infectious. My presence put people at risk, and this made me feel self-conscious. The same feelings, reactions, thoughts and perceptions I felt as that rejected, rebellious child, surfaced again. I thought it would be easier to go through this experience if I pushed everyone away and resurrected the carefully assembled barriers of yesteryear.

My communication skills were inadequate. I didn't understand what I was feeling. Deep down, I knew my thoughts were irrational and negative, but I didn't possess the skills or knowledge to change them or seek support. I could yell, deflect and manipulate, but actually talk? Well, that just wasn't me. I thought it would be easier for me to negotiate the rapids of this journey alone.

I knew I could weather the storm. I had done it before. History had equipped me with skills to persevere. I would draw on these skills and apply them to this situation. I deliberately turned my face away from John, and turned to face the fierce wind alone.

> *"Determination and perseverance move the world; thinking that others will do it for you is a sure way to fail."*
>
> *Marva Collins*

Chapter 41

Defeated by thoughts

"Sow a thought, and you reap an act; Sow an act, and you reap a habit; Sow a habit, and you reap a character; Sow a character, and you reap a destiny."
- Charles Reade

My mind just wouldn't give up. Horror stories depicting sinister and catastrophic events engulfed me. Isolated, lonely and friendless scenarios flowed like honey through my mind, coating and sticking to every curve and fissure. Whispered expressions of devastation constantly tinkled in my ears. They warned me of my husband's withdrawal and pending departure.

Unanswered questions constantly blazed like luminescent words on a billboard. Why would he want to stay in this marriage? What would possess him to stay with me? I believed I was an infected, ugly piece of human flesh. Why would he want to be with me? I ruminated about him living an alternative life. My fears and doubts about myself and the family rose with every new day.

Continuous insecurities dominated my thinking. They superseded all other thoughts, and triggered and produced pessimistic, melancholy scenarios in every situation I found myself in. I thought I was highly infectious, which caused me to become paranoid that I might infect someone and made me withdraw even more.

Daily, the internal black hole, which had now taken up residence within me, fought to consume me. I continually struggled against its rising tide of despair, but often lost the skirmish to fall deeply into the unfathomable void of depression that lay waiting to ensnare me. I couldn't see a way out. There was no light to direct me. My own pride prevented me from allowing the people who mattered in my life to actually see what was happening to me. I forced myself to live in a cycle of regret, distress, self-loathing and isolation. My thoughts and fears of infecting another crippled me. I wrestled often with these thoughts and fought hard not to be dragged down their treacherous path, but my mind was so weak. What if it was one of my children, even a stranger? No, I could never let that happen. I would leave before I would let myself be a part of that scenario.

Every night I would lie in my bed, with the warmth of my husband's body against my back, his face snuggled into my neck, and every day I would fearfully open my eyes, and think, today is the day. John would make the decision to end it. He needed a better life. I would simply let him go. I would not struggle or force him to stay, for I knew it was the best solution. But, surprisingly, each day he would stay, and I would question and speculate why.

Faceless demons never left my side, they continued to taunt me. Sometimes they grew stronger, consumed my thoughts, sometimes they changed direction and hit me from another angle, but they were ever present and constant in their pursuit to destroy me.

I hated the way I was feeling. I just couldn't seem to shake the feelings of hopelessness which burned me, or the misery and sadness that plagued me. How was I ever going to recover from this? I wondered if I would ever see a crack in the never ending tunnel that had encircled my life.
I was always so driven to achieve. I had overcome adversity before, I just could not work out why this challenge was so different.

"An oak and a reed were arguing about their strength. When a strong wind came up, the reed avoided being uprooted by bending and leaning with the gusts of wind. But the oak stood firm and was torn up by the roots".

Aesop

Chapter 42

Personal reflection

I now realise that I was probably suffering from depression. Up until this point, I didn't really know what depression was. I had no experience with it, but this situation gave me a true look at the nature of depression and how easily it can rob you of your life. It can consume every part of you. It slowly creeps into your life and steals your sanity. Like a thief in the night, it calmly strips you bare, until you believe there is absolutely nothing left; no hope, no way out. All is lost. The pit is so deep, so dark, so consuming and so easily accepted.

What I didn't understand, until much later, was that my false perceptions changed how I thought, how I acted and behaved and this altered all my relationships and my interactions, and all in such a short time. My relationship with John went from being stable and healthy to being unstable and unhealthy in a matter of weeks. Living with and believing all my negative perceptions changed how I interacted with everyone. My perceptions sabotaged my life and prevented me from reaching out to people who wanted to help me. My attitudes and behaviours based on these perceptions caused major rifts to form between myself, my family, and my friends. The act of withdrawing from everyone pushed the people I needed most further away from me. What I should have done was to share my fears with them, so they could understand what was happening to me. But I didn't.

> *"If you do what you've always done, you'll get what you've always gotten."*
>
> *Anthony Robbins*

Chapter 43

Family loyalty

"The purpose of life is a life of purpose."
~Robert Byrne

I allowed a tornado with two spouts, called my diagnosis, to abruptly rise from the depths of my life, and annihilation and chaos came with it. Within three short weeks, the foster world I thought I intimately knew became entangled in a vortex and spiralled out of my control, removing everything that had grounded me over the last 20 years.

My sex life became non-existent. Any intimate moments we shared were shrouded in a veil of masked, deep-seated fear. How could I be intimate with my husband? What if I infected him? I didn't know how to act 'normally' around him anymore, especially in the bedroom. Before my diagnosis, we had enjoyed a very active sex life. I didn't know if I could continue that now. Did I even want to? No, I would not put him at risk. I made a choice, and I withdrew that as well, which left very little to base our relationship on.

Surely now, it would end. He would move on. I knew this would break my heart, but I was prepared, for I believed it was inevitable and the best thing for everyone. I loved him deeply, even in my dysfunctional state. He was a kind, caring, reliable man. A rock I could stand on in times of need. I knew staying with me was essentially a dangerous, and potentially deadly, prospect for him, and I believed it would be better if it all ended.

However, he again didn't leave like I expected. He chose to stand beside me. A decision I did not fully understand. There was no real basis to this, our new relationship, but the root of time and the years of shared experiences. A Hep C tsunami had struck its hardest blow and our foundations had been severely shaken, yet our love still stood. Why? I kept asking myself. Why was he still with me? Could he love me that much that he would risk his life to be with me? This though shocked me...

I closely watched him as he processed everything that was happening around him, but still he stood firm. His unwavering dedication to our relationship changed how I perceived him. I started to really look at him, and I saw a very different man than I had first married. I saw subtle changes that I had never seen before, probably because I was always so self-absorbed and career focussed. I'd never really looked at him. He had matured, grown, and I had missed the process. It was then that I realised I didn't see things how they really were. I saw our relationship and life as I was. John had become a strong person, full of conviction and loyalty to his family, and I hadn't seen this man before. I thought, if he believed in us this much, then I needed to pull myself together, and start to fight as well. Fight, for not only my life, but for the family unit I had once helped to create.

"Dreams are only an indication of what you can do, but a burning desire combined with action is the way to live its reality."

Byron Pulsifer

Chapter 44

My internal pain
"I am an example to many people, because you are my strong protection."
Psalm 71:7

During the initial stages of my diagnosis, the GP advised us to get John tested. We were told I potentially could have infected him over our twenty years together. The thought of this scenario crushed me. It was a blow to my spirit that I just didn't need right now. The time between the test and the results passed so agonizingly slowly, and it was the grimmest of times for me. Guilt and blame assaulted me from every angle. I perceived John would blame me and further reject me, and if I had indeed infected him, this would be the first nail in my coffin, and the lid would slam shut nice and tight, snuffing out my life in the process.

The agonising wait was over. The results were in. We drove to the surgery, five kilometres from our home. The air in the car was heavy with our thoughts. I turned my face to look out the passenger window, silently allowing the tears to fill my eyes and gently fall down my cheeks. Words can't explain what I felt at that moment. It was one of the bleakest days I had witnessed, filled with fear, regret and dread.

We sat together quietly, on the cold plastic chairs. The flurry and commotion of the busy surgery surrounded and distracted us. I wanted to be in some other alternate reality, something out of the Twilight Zone, or the Fringe. A reality I was not really in, but could observe from the outside. Young children with snotty noses and crusty eyes peered at us from the safety and security of their mother's side. A TV boomed non-descript daily news directly above us, phones constantly rung and people steadily moved in and out of doctors' rooms. The all-encompassing noise and movement was stifling, yet somehow, comforting in its diversion from my predicament.

The doctor's door opened. There he stood. He looked at John and me, as we nervously waited, with compassion and understanding. He raised his hand, and beckoned us into his oversized, cluttered room. For the first time in days, my husband grabbed my hand. I turned to look up at him, my dazed and saddened blue eyes filled with tears.

He eyes sunk into mine. Time stood still. His pale green eyes pierced straight into my soul, reading every thought and feeling I had. My heavily burdened heart pounded furiously in my chest. I was nervous and scared, wondering what he would say to me. My eyes moved to look at his half open, upturned mouth as his eyes were too intense for me to focus upon. He slowly leaned closer to me, his lips grazed my ear. His whispered words resonated in my mind and stilled the negative dialogue within me, "it is going to be alright, Laurie."

I was still unsure. Had I infected him? I would know within minutes. How would he react if the test was positive? Would he hate me? Would this terminate our relationship? How would I react? What would happen to the children if both of us were infected? What had I done, all those years ago? Look what those actions had produced all these years later? How could I have been so stupid, so selfish?

I unsteadily got up from the chair and slowly turned towards the door. My feet automatically, yet reluctantly, moved me, my trendy blue Nike runners felt like heavy pieces of concrete attached to my feet. What a predicament I had placed us in! The situation was completely surreal. As I reached the door, I recalled my husband's words and his simple captivating smile, "It is going to be alright." Did he truly mean those words? I don't know if I would feel the same if I found myself in his shoes. Would I feel the same? I doubted it.

His strength of character, a mighty power which shone from him, its potency and intensity, totally absorbed me. Could there possibly be a fracture in the outer lining of the dark tunnel which encircled me? Was it possible to see a glimmer of light and hope? Was John strong enough to carry both of us through this? I thought he just might be.

We sat in the chairs and faced the doctor who had been our GP for the last eight years. He knew all our history. He had always dealt with us in his non-judgmental, kind and compassionate nature, and today would be no different. He was someone who we had grown to care for and trust over the years.

This was our moment, a defining moment, unmercifully suspended. I felt like a prisoner on death row, awaiting my sentence; my pending mortal punishment for the life I chose. This was the very last moment before judgment reigned upon me. The doctor sympathetically scrutinized both of us, then asked how we were. I looked at him astonished. Words failed me. I thought, if you only knew the weight of the burdens we carried! I knew he was genuinely concerned about our situation, but every delay was an agonizing blow to me. I just wanted to yell "hurry up! Give us the results!" I answered his question with a simple nod, my eyes drawn to the computer screen, where I knew the answer lay waiting to be revealed. My fingers fidgeted, busy, as they annoyed a piece of fabric on the hem of my shorts.

Finally, the computer screen jumped to life. John's medical history opened up in front of me, pages containing columns of facts and figures, unlocked for me to see. I leant forward. My eyes furiously scanned the information as it unravelled. I searched only for what I truly needed: a result, a simple positive or negative.
The doctor sat quietly as he discerned the results. Finally he turned to face us. His deep brown eyes peered over the top of his silver rimmed spectacles. He paused, and then turned the old computer screen towards us to allow us to see the data on the screen. Old historical appointments and outcomes filled the page, so much information, it was impossible for me to distinguish the results.

John's green eyes jumped from the doctor to the screen and back again. I knew he was trying desperately to detect and recognise something. His eyes finally settled unemotionally on the doctor, waiting. My impatience and anxiety grew, it growled inside me, threatening to eat up my determination to sit quietly. He finally spoke, directing all his words to the man who sat calmly and intently beside me. His eyes never left John's face, his full attention channelled towards him. The hammer hit the anvil. It delivered its verdict. Two sets of eyes now penetrated and probed me for a response. I felt the heat of their glances as they searched and questioned me, interested in my reaction to the outcome.

I sat stunned as my mind tried to rationalise the result. How could that be? He was negative, but, how? What did this mean? I never considered that to be a possibility. Of course, I wanted him to have this kind of outcome, but I never believed it would be possible. It was unimaginable, unreal, remarkable and awesome. I felt humbled by this result. Humbled that I could be given another chance. Humbled that I had not infected him and humbled that he still loved me, after all of this.

All of a sudden, my mind filled with hundreds of questions, as they all fought to be heard. How could this be? What sort of infectious disease was this? I recalled some risky situations we had been in during our marriage, where my blood had come in contact with his, and still he was not infected. How come? I started to see a glimmer of real, tangible hope. I could see a fracture in the tunnel wall and a tiny ray of light beamed steadily in the darkness. A lifeline was offered, a rope to guide me, and I gladly received it. However, I wondered if it would be sturdy enough to save me before the walls collapsed under the weight of the burdens I carried. Was there now a possibility of some hope for us? Could we actually live together without a constant threat lurking in the background? If so, I wouldn't have to leave. Was that a possibility?

The air seemed to collapse around me, sucked out by an overpowered vacuum, and replaced with a beautiful, sweet aroma. My stiffness and tension were erased by a few simple words, "not infected." Relaxation crept into my being, like a slow rising mist. A symphony played soothing notes, its calming effects flowed over me.

My senses were alert, sharpened by this new situation. I sat silently evaluating John's reaction. After twenty years of marriage, I could identify minute, but subtle, changes in him. Small, unseen gestures, slight changes in his tone of voice and minor body movements, detected by me, but unrecognisable to others. I waited quietly, intimately trying to decipher his signals. John's face beamed like the sun. Joy radiated from him. He was genuinely happy, relieved by the news, and so was I.

Would I now be able to lay to rest some of the unspeakable guilt that burdened me daily? Could I possibly offload and be free from some of my own convictions? I knew none of this would equate to absolution. But could I really find relief and be rid of some of my guilt? Was it a possibility? I had not infected him. This fact brought hope with it.

As I looked at the people before me, I said a silent prayer of thanks to a God I only slightly knew.
I had not been really close to God. I knew of Him, I had witnessed things and had firsthand experience of His capabilities, but I didn't really know Him. I guess I was what you would call, "a Clayton's Christian," an on-again-off-again kind of person who practised the principles only when it suited me. However, I knew very well what He was capable of doing. I just never really believed that the promises in the Bible applied to me, as I was so sinful; unworthy in every respect of the word. So, why would He want to help someone like me? But right now, I felt He did, and I couldn't be more grateful.

Walking out of that medical centre, towards the waiting car, I felt like I wanted to kiss the hard concrete surface that my unencumbered feet walked upon. The euphoria and relief this forecast brought was a turning point for both of us. We were united in hope, and together, we had overcome our first major milestone. We also knew many more hardship lay before us, threatening us. But, as we left that building, we were a silhouette of a happy couple.

We held hands, content and delighted, both of us encouraged by the results. This victory made us believe the journey stretching out in front of us would be worth the fight. We decided today we would savour the victory and revel in its glory, cherishing and committing the moment to memory, for tomorrow was a new day and an ominous, snow-covered mountain loomed before us, and we both knew that the hardest path was yet to come.

"Out of a hundred years a few minutes were made that stayed with me, not a hundred years".
~Antonio Porchia,

Chapter 45

Attitude is everything
"The fear of life is the favourite disease of the 20th century."
*~**William Lyon Phelps***

The days that followed John's clearance were filled with more optimism. My overall perception and outlook for our future changed after that message of hope. Positive notes, affirmation and images started to spice up my mind and replaced some of the negative undertones. Their essence infused anticipation and overrode the acid flavours of the recent past.

I don't know why, but I started to pray more regularly. I believed I had been given a sign when John's test came back negative. I only hoped it wasn't a one-time thing, because I was seeking help again. My daily prayer, "God, I know I am unworthy to come before you, but I am here asking for your help. Please hear me. I need to be healed. I know I doubt you have a purpose for my life, help me to understand why this is happening to me and help me see the good in all of this."

Changes appeared subtly, they crept into my life slowly. I found I was focussing more on positive things, and I became more optimistic. After a while, I could visualise a hopeful future full of expectations. To maintain this, I constantly had to have the right attitude, an attitude of faith, forgiveness, love and hope. This was a hard feat for anyone to maintain, especially when the dark passenger lurked in the background.

My previous self-destructive beliefs and attitude had shackled me in the past. I could not allow them to confine or blind me anymore. Our recent good news, as well as the realisation that John was not going anywhere, had released me from the chains which prevented me from positively engaging in my life. I wanted and needed to return emotionally, physically and psychologically to my marriage.

My self-imposed dark pit was no longer as ominous or as deep as I had imagined. I could see the top, and I started to claw my way up, out towards the daylight. I dug deep into the hard clay to ensure a strong foot hold as I manoeuvred out of the mess my life had become. I would fight back. I wanted a life, a future with John. I would not roll over and let this disease rob me of everything I cared about. It had already stolen weeks of my life, nearly destroying me in the process. I would not lie down and let it kick me again.

Once my attitude started to change and I started to fight for what was already mine, I was surprised to discover how deeply and sincerely I was loved. John demonstrated his undying love for me time and time again, I was just too blind to see it or accept it. If John had the guts to stay with me, standing stoically beside me, unwavering in his conviction, then I would not give up. I would fight, and fight damn hard, for my life.

I vowed to learn everything I could about my hidden passenger, and banish it from my life. I chose to pick up my weapons of war. My steel armour would be created from the knowledge I would gain. I would protect my heart and my mind using the love of my family to support me. A helmet of faith would adorn my head to help me combat the mental attacks that regularly plagued me. The treatment I would hopefully access would be my sword and deliver the final blow and rid me of HCV forever.

"Be kinder than necessary, for everyone you meet is fighting some kind of battle"

- Author unknown

Chapter 46

Formulating a battle strategy

"It is a common experience that a problem difficult at night is resolved in the morning after the committee of sleep has worked on it."
~John Steinbeck

HCV resembled Mount Everest. I stood at its base and looked up as I tried to plot the best and safest path I should take to conquer this ominous disease. I decided to systematically examine, investigate and analyse it, so I could better understand the situation I was in. I chose to assess the history of HCV, its capabilities, its strengths and weakness, and how it was cured.

This tiny body snatcher, my unknown invader for the last 20 years, was totally immersed in my life substance. Its venom saturated my blood. It was my co-host, a being I shared my body with daily. Until now, we had lived in some sort of harmony. An unknown compromise had been reached between my body and this virus; a cycle only my immune system understood, and one my mind wanted liberation from. To do this, I knew my body had to become inhospitable to this virus, and to make that happen I needed to totally understand the mysterious, microscopic passenger I had picked up.

Over the next few months, I found myself enthusiastically consumed with internet research. Page after page devoted to suitable, consistent information. I was interested in everything: conflicting views, treatments, natural therapies, medical journals, blogs and testimonials. I hungered for it all, devoured and gorged myself on their substance, like a ravenous wolf.

I began to feel in control, the scales now weighed in my favour. Learning enabled me to slowly assess the terrain of Mount Everest and formulate a skilled strategy to start my climb. Wisdom replaced my ignorance. As I grew in both knowledge and awareness, I became less vulnerable to the attacks of my darker side. I learnt to deflect the whispering voices and the harmful messages and replace them with wisdom. This wisdom brought forth maturity and growth within me.

I finally stopped feeling sorry for myself, and ceased to blame others for the things of the past. I realised I was accountable, and I took responsibility for what I had done, no longer making excuses for my poor behaviour. I realised that no one talked me into doing anything. I chose to participate, and I did so willingly, so the blame was at my feet, no one else's. I could now accept that.

I also grew stronger in my faith, and I learnt to accept my life and what I had been given. I started to believe in the promises which were previously explained to me by Sue all those years ago. I found that as I took this path it strengthened me.
I hope you find something to help you on your life's path. For me, I found God. I found something I could hold onto, something I could trust. Believing helped me understand. It helped me forgive. It helped me learn to love and trust again, and made me feel a part of something special.

I believe all our lives are special in their own unique way. We need to accept the things of the past and make the best of what lies ahead. Our circumstances are temporary but our character is not.

"There are very few human beings who receive the truth, complete and staggering, by instant illumination. Most of them acquire it fragment by fragment, on a small scale, by successive developments, cellularly, like a laborious mosaic."

~Anaïs Nin

Chapter 47

Nothing in life truly remains hidden
"Diseases can be our spiritual flat tires - disruptions in our lives that seem to be disasters at the time but end by redirecting our lives in a meaningful way".
~Bernie S. Siegel

My specialist appointment was only a few short weeks away. I had waited apprehensively for three and a half, long-drawn-out months to see this man. I hoped he would help me. I had reams and reams of data I had collated and tried to interpret. Two large folders were filled with information on managing my disease, natural treatments and treatment options. I knew from the information I had collected that the Pegasys brand of interferon and ribavirn held a better cure rate, so I hoped he would endorse that product. I also had compiled a long list of questions, and, hopefully his answers would dispel some of my internal fears.

Up until this point, only John and I were aware of my infection. We had not informed anyone, but before I saw the specialist, I knew we had to inform the family. We couldn't leave it much longer. John and I were resilient, but their suffering was something neither of us wanted to witness. My study had equipped us with an armoury of answers to respond to the questions when the time came.

I was reticent to uncover any of my past to those closest to me, especially the portions I had tried to forget. I had discarded my old life a long time ago, burying it in a steel casket. I also didn't like that decayed person, and I certainly wasn't keen to revisit my past. But, here I was, forced to revive it. I was nothing like that old rotting corpse. I was reborn. I lived a vastly different lifestyle now. My recollections of this old life were both distasteful and confronting. I could see no honour or esteem in any of it.

My diagnosis made me realise nothing in life stays completely hidden or remains in the darkness forever. It seems that everything is eventually revealed, uncovered, brought out into the open, for the whole world to see, whether you like it or not. This was my moment, my revelation. Back then, I didn't think about the consequences of any of my actions, but I was not so naive today. My penalty had caused so much anguish, sorrow and embarrassment to myself and to John, and now I had to face the children.

I felt uncomfortable and humiliated in this situation. There was no way out, but to tell the truth. They needed to hear the whole truth, and they would. I vowed to withhold nothing from them. If they asked a question, I would honestly and openly answer it. I knew it would be hard, but I also knew I had to forge a path forward, and this was just one of those critical and essential steps I needed to take.

We had excluded them for months as we pretended and covered our anguish with a blanket of invented happiness. I am not really sure why we did this. Maybe we both were in a form of denial, trying to forget about it. I believed we needed to find a sense of peace with each other, as well as understand our feelings and the impact HCV had on our marriage, before we could talk about it to others. Time enabled us to assess the situation, and provided us with a breathing space to accept what had happened. The stability of our future relationship was my main reason for the delay. I only hoped the family would understand my reasons and could accept the fact that we had needed this time.

"When I stand before God at the end of my life, I would hope that I would not have a single bit of talent left, and could say, "I used everything you gave me."

~Erma Bombeck

Chapter 48

Asking the hard questions
"In ordinary life we hardly realize that we receive a great deal more than we give, and that it is only with gratitude that life becomes rich."
- Dietrich Bonhoeffer

John and I still needed to discuss our feelings and work out a solid plan for the future so we could offer the kids a solution when we spoke to them.

We sat together on the patio which overlooked the pebbled concrete pool. The sweet aroma of coffee floated gently around us on the delicate breeze, the sun was high in the sky, its rays sparkled on the rippling surface of the pool as we both sipped our hot beverages. We sat comfortably in the deck chairs, enjoying the moment, conscious that a serious, in-depth conversation was pending.

My main concern was how he felt about sharing a life and living in close proximity with someone in my condition. I knew he had previously stated he was with me until the end, but we had both had time to process the situation, and we really had not discussed any of our fears.

I was nervous about the responses he may offer to my questions. However, I hoped he would be truly honest. I needed the truth to gauge the state of our relationship, and, our future. I also wanted to have some time to discuss the treatment options and his risk factors. I knew if I was able to summarize what I had learnt, it would reassure him. His risks were minimal, negligible even, but he needed to believe that. We started our conversation by deliberating his negative result, both of us amazed and happy he was not infected.

We casually talked about all the medical journals I had uncovered. I had identified how we could prevent transmission between us. It was simple. We just couldn't share any of my toiletries like my razor, tweezers or any other item that may have my blood on it. We would also need to be more vigilant about open wounds, and having unprotected sex during my period. We also talked in length about the Pegasys treatment, its cure rates, natural therapies, and what could possibly happen to me.

We talked for hours. We shared our feelings, our fears, our hopes, and together, we cried.

Our sex life was a component of this relationship, which I was nervous to explore. I posed my question, how did he feel about having sex with me, now that I was infectious? I really just wanted to know if he feared becoming infected. His answer was slow to come. His eyes were cagey and unable to focus on mine. Finally, they settled on the surface of the pool. He was noticeably edgy, fidgeting with his cold, nearly empty coffee mug. He was voiceless, for a long moment. His unfocussed eyes stared, but did not genuinely see anything. I think he processed internal words I guessed he would never say.

I am not sure, but, I sincerely think he wanted to say yes, he feared becoming infected. Never the less, he graciously didn't. How would I have reacted if he had? I really don't know. Thankfully, I didn't have to deal with that scenario. I am sure that if I heard the words I thought I was going to hear, I might have plummeted headfirst back into the pit I had fought so strongly to avoid. His negative answer would have most definitely affected our ongoing relationship. I was glad he lied. I realised I didn't really want to hear the truth. He had the maturity and the forward thinking to understand what the truth might have done to us, so he kept his thought to himself. One day I may ask him if my perception was correct.

"Some luck lies in not getting what you thought you wanted but getting what you have, which once you have got it you may be smart enough to see is what you would have wanted had you known."

~Garrison Keillor

Chapter 49

A panoramic view
"The best and most beautiful things in this world cannot be seen or even heard, but must be felt with the heart".
- Helen Keller

Even though I felt more settled, I found it impossible to make any future plans. My perception that I may not have long to live prevented this from occurring. I understood the risk and protective factors, but I didn't know how the disease had affected me personally. What if I had cirrhosis or serious liver damage? For now, I thought it was easier and wiser to live in the moment and not plan or think about what tomorrow may hold.

At times my life didn't feel real. I felt like a fictional character in an elusive story. Life seemed to move completely out of my control, and I sometimes felt like a spectator watching as scenarios manipulated by someone else played out before me.

In the back of my mind, I was haunted by the prospect that someone else was in charge of my destiny, and the realisation that I could be taken from this earth at anytime. I came to believe that our days are numbered. I theorised that our death is predestined, the date already written by our Creator. Finding myself in this situation made me confront and accept my own mortality.

It made me think, maybe life was a bit like a performance review, assessing our behaviours and attitudes, then providing correction. It sometimes felt like it. I know my own internal broadcasting system regularly reminded me of my poor behaviour and attitude.

I explained to John, I wished for a time machine, to go back and undo what I did all those years ago, to save us both from this experience and all the painful events to come. I also talked about my constant self-doubt and self-questioning. I wondered why we were going through this, and why now? What I didn't realise, until our talk, was that he asked himself the same questions.

During our talk, I uncovered all my inner feelings, my uncertainties and my reservations. All my cards lay on the table, exposed to this man, the man I had married over 20 years ago. I laid the inner parts of myself out before him, something I had never done before. They were an offering at the altar of our marriage for him to accept or reject. There was no turning back now. I wondered what he would think of me now that he was aware of the darkness that sometimes rose up within me. He was now aware of the voices that had lived within me all these years, undermining my self-esteem.

I felt our talk was one of the first tangible steps we took, together, towards really managing my HCV.

Those hours spent by the pool that day sincerely connected us. They opened my eyes to his concerns and personal fears, as well as enabled me to see the real man I was married to. I really saw the changes in him that day. He was transformed. His sympathy for my plight and his pure determination to stand by me boosted my commitment to overcome this speed bump. As I listened to him speak, my loyalty and devotion to our relationship strengthened.

A new alliance formed between us. It grew stronger each day. It fostered courage, support and most of all, love. I learnt a major lesson that day; one that altered the deeply rooted conscripts which surrounded my life, and all my old belief systems were converted.

What stunned me the most was just how easy it was to talk to him, to tell him how I felt. I was able to rationalise my thoughts without any judgment, condemnation or criticism, and I was able to listen to his enlightening responses. I was embraced, surrounded by tenderness, not blamed, just loved and accepted. I had discovered someone I could really trust. This level of communication, had never occurred between us ever before, and it felt good.

His words throughout the conversation implied that he did want to stay with me, and he did trust me. He stated he was in this marriage for the long haul and would not throw the towel in now, just because of a slight rough patch we faced. Our marriage vows were permanently imprinted on his heart. He had said yes to "in sickness and in health" and he chose to support me through this battle. I wanted to believe all of his words, but the dark passenger's whispered doubts, full of scepticism, rose.

Words are meaningless, empty and futile unless they are backed by real, decisive action. This was a tough situation for him to be in. Tough decisions lay before him. I was infectious, and he was not infected. Sex put him at risk. Even if it was a miniscule risk, it was still a threat; it would be a constant hazard in our relationship. In his mind, I would imagine, it was like playing Russian roulette, a game of probability, every time he thought about sleeping with me. He never discussed this aspect, or his feelings around this issue, but his short period of personal withdrawal conveyed his uncertainty.

I think his physical, primal desires overrode the psychological dangers, as we did finally resume a normal sex life. It wasn't the sex I had missed so much, but I needed to feel wanted, needed and loved. A simple touch, a slight brush of the hand, a stroke of the hair, or a simple loving look says more than words ever can, and I had missed these.

"Who will tell whether one happy moment of love or the joy of breathing or walking on a bright morning and smelling the fresh air, is not worth all the suffering and effort which life implies"

~Erich Fromm

Chapter 50

A one way trip
"Some people are born into wonderful families. Others have to find or create them. Being a member of a family is a priceless membership that we pay nothing for but love."
- Jim Stovall

A few days elapsed after our talk, and we both felt confident and comfortable enough to talk to the children. The night before our big reveal, I found it impossible to sleep. A violent storm raged within me. I was like a ship, tossed in the throes of a tormented sea, unable to be stilled. I got up from my bed and paced the kitchen whilst wordless pantomimes, with faceless actors, performed my unspoken fears on a stage only I could see. Phrase less, pessimistic and destructive words sprawled across the theatre walls, like huge, seductive streamers. What were the right words to use? How would I deliver them? The answers refused to come. I prayed long and hard, to seek guidance, and finally, I found peace, and rest fell upon me.

Our children, the oldest, my daughter, reminded me of the sun. She possesses a natural charismatic beauty. A warmth and vitality blaze from her. The energy she emits supports and influences the life around her. My youngest was more like the earth. He retains incredible depth and power. His words carry multi-layered meaning and profound thought. He possesses fierce intensity and diversity, as well as resilience to overcome and change a reactive environment.

Our family life and the seasonal changes we all experienced were governed by the deep connection between these two children. The sun had nurtured and provided light to the earth when the storms of life had struck. They drew on each other's strengths, supported and encouraged each other in times of trouble, and I hoped their alliance would help them in the tough times that lay ahead.

The four of us together made up our own unique planet. A planet only we understood and felt comfortable in; one where we shared creation, development, history and affection. Our lives were perpetually intertwined, and I trusted this would not change after they heard my story.

My love for my children surged like the rapids of a waterfall. The powerful emotions I felt for them engulfed, embraced and accepted everything they did. I could not lose either of them. My sole purpose was to preserve the peaceful and calm waters of the environment we currently lived in. My wish, like any protective mother, was that my words would not cause either of them distress or pain. I just wanted them to continue to positively grow and prosper, not to be burdened, with my worries. Their lives held enough of their own challenges, and setbacks as they travelled their own course through life.

I believe life is but a succession of moments; a one way trip. I had one shot at this. I knew every word spoken could never be taken back. So I needed to be mindful and choose my words carefully, in an attempt to make the children feel as secure as possible as we told them.

Both their lives had just begun. Their paths were still being crafted. I did not want my words to extinguish all that we had formed over the years. If this trust was lost, it could cut a path of destruction in all of our lives. Trust is a fragile concept, something that can be lost in an instance. The last thing I wanted was for the kids to start to erect negative and destructive strongholds in their lives like I did as a child.

I also didn't want to betray either of my children by being deceitful or dishonest. I hoped their hearts would not harden at my words or their backs turn towards me. I would speak honestly, openly, and with a true heart, to both of them. I would not walk in the shadows anymore. I vowed to try and endure this situation, and everything else that would occur, from this point on, with as much grace and dignity as I possessed.

> *"Look not mournfully into the past, it comes not back again. Wisely improve the present, it is thine. Go forth to meet the shadowy future without fear and with a manly heart."*
>
> ***Henry Wadsworth Longfellow***

Chapter 51
The innocence of children
"A journey may be long or short, but it must start at the very spot one finds oneself."
- Jim Stovall

My youngest still lived at home with John and I. He was a fourteen-year-old young man, who possessed innocence and an openness to experience the unbound world, he lived in. His life required simple needs, such as time, and a comfortable space to grow. His current youthful journey was without destination; no plans had been set. I was about to disrupt his world and potentially create an unstable and turbulent time for him.

I had never spoken of my past to him, so he was unknown to the challenging world in which I grew up. However, he was about to be enlightened to the girl who lay under the mask. I wondered how he would react. Would he withdraw, unable to understand, or would he accept my previous life choices? I hoped he would be able to understand that everything I did back then was done when I was living a different life in difficult circumstances, a life before he was born. I was scared of losing his love. It would cause a pain no medicine would ever cure. My life would become a windowless, cold, empty, dark room if he withdrew from me.

I knew the words I had to say were going to ruin the well-built, secure and safe structures that supported his world. His life was already in unfamiliar territory. He had recently experienced a change in schools, the loss of all his childhood school friends and familiar surroundings, add to that hormonal changes, and now this! How would he cope?

His melancholy nature meant he was analytical, thoughtful, and very thorough. Detailed, perhaps is a better word. At times he could appear completely unenthusiastic, but I knew he just needed to understand the purpose behind the task. All of this aside, I found him to be self-sacrificing and extraordinarily loyal.

I knew that it would be crucial to take a detailed approach with him, one that was succinct and supported by literature. I would also need to be optimistic, supportive and have a planned approach towards a positive outcome, one he could understand. He needed details, and I would provide them to him so he could contemplate and ruminate over them. The last thing I wanted was to trigger a negative emotional response in him, such as fear or depression. Even though I was quite thorough in my planning ability, I doubted my own emotional capability to pull it off, without causing him undue distress.

'Never tell people how to do things. Tell them what to do and they will surprise you with their ingenuity.'

George Patton

Chapter 52

Words from Heaven fall
"A flower has to go through a lot of dirt before it can bloom."
- ***Author unknown***

I set what I considered to be the right scene. I cooked a succulent roast beef dinner, with browned, crunchy-baked potatoes, served with mounds of emerald green peas and moist, juicy corn; his favourite meal. Together, we sat at the table, each of us awkwardly toying with our food. An arctic fog of apprehension slowly swirled around each of us, our thoughts frozen. Silence lingered and hung heavily in the air. We waited for the first words to cut through the icy environment.

My mind focused on trying to create those respectable first words. I genuinely couldn't start the conversation, as the right words wouldn't form. I heard hushed words as they echoed around the room. They rebounded off John, and rung steadily in my ears. "What is this all about? What is going on? You guys have been weird for ages." His questions were like a boomerang, circling in my head, unable to return to its original thrower.

My eyes were unable to touch my son's inquisitive face, for fear of his rejection if he saw what my face portrayed. My heavy heart lifted its pace, ready for the race ahead. My lungs battled for more breath to accommodate its pace. My frustrated mind tried to process his questions. It sought answers in an abyss of unusable words.

I placed my fork next to my untouched, gravy-covered meat. I searched John's face for reassurance and assistance. A flood of salty tears quickly pooled, then gently fell over my eye lids and tumbled down my cheeks. I seldom cried in front of the children, so this action made my son extremely edgy and uneasy. He shrieked, "What is going on?" My voice vanished, trapped in the void between invention and expression, leaving John to explain our predicament, as I mutely wept. Through my tears, I searched his face, hunting for any sign of reassurance that he understood, and that he was going to be okay.

Moments passed. I slowly regained my composure, my voice soft, but full of conviction. I offered him detailed information regarding HCV, and how we planned to rise above and triumph over this difficulty that faced us. I explained I had an appointment with the specialist in a few weeks and we would know more then.

He became very still, very silent, a fourteen-year-old boy in emotional turmoil, processing, adding another problem to his life. He swivelled the steel dinner fork between his thumb and forefinger, and teased a lone green pea, obviously preoccupied with the content of our conversation. Unexpectedly, he stood up, staggered slightly, found his balance, and then left the room, his dinner hardly touched. His silent withdrawal from the table left John and I speechless. He entered his room, slipped between the sheets of his double bed, and refused to communicate or socialise with either of us for the next two days.

What a predicament I found myself in! A predicament I knew I had brought upon us. This situation was entirely my fault. My sinister passenger thrashed within me. It flung debris at me from every angle. The wreckage of my previous choices struck me from every side, leaving me incapacitated by their force. What had I done to this family? What had I done to myself? Could I ever redeem myself? Somehow, I doubted it. My existence threatened everyone. I wanted to escape. Even a small diversion from the reality of all of this would help. But, I felt so tethered, completely bound to the unfolding situation. I wanted to be that free horse that raced over the distant hill, the one from my childhood imagination, not this restrained, tightly reigned mount.

What could I possibly do to help him? His needs totally escaped me. I didn't know what to do. I wanted to take away his pain; the pain I knew I had caused. I would take it all, if I could. What sort of mother was I, to do this to a child whom I loved more than life itself?

I believed no-one could possibly understand the heavy yoke I carried, or the toll this all took on my life. I wouldn't talk about these feelings to anyone. I couldn't. I wouldn't let any of my family see this vulnerable side of me. They relied on me to be the strong one, and that was what I would try and portray. But, if they only knew what was really going on inside me, I think they would be shocked. In reality, I felt weak, pathetic and undeserving to be a part of this family.

I left the table and stood outside, alone. Tears clouded my eyes as I stood on the patio. Through the watery veil I could see the brilliant glow of the moon as it floated in the cloudless night. Stars shone vibrantly overhead, and the entire landscape before me was illuminated. I knew I needed time to think, but trying to see through the thick mud my gloomy thoughts had created was nearly impossible.

As I looked up at the moon through my blurry eyes, it dawned on me that the moon had no light of its own. It just reflects the brilliance and radiance of another planet, the sun. A thought dropped into my mind. This was exactly what I had to learn to do. If I was to survive this ride, I needed to reflect more confidence and enthusiasm. I had to borrow the skills of my old friend the chameleon and reflect positivism and optimism. I simply couldn't let the family see the pit I continually cycled in and out of. It would scare them, just as it scared me.

I knew I needed to stop all the negative thoughts that plagued me. I had already successfully learnt how to change the negative visual pictures and replace them with brighter, more affirming, positive and constructive images. This practice had helped to some extent. But in times like this, I found it nearly impossible to rewrite any new scripts. My feelings of immorality and self-loathing were so strong, they overrode any skills I had previously learnt.

I would need to engage in a personal battle, an internal war, with my own mind; one I dared not lose, if I wanted to help my family. I identified that I couldn't help them if I was not able to overcome the conflict that wrestled constantly within me. I simply couldn't keep coming back to the same place every time something went wrong.

However, my emotions were so fragile, so up and down, it was hard to focus on anything positive whilst my son lay in his bed and suffered. But, I knew I had to stop this cyclic behaviour. It was completely unhealthy, not only for me, but for the rest of the family

I also comprehended that I simply couldn't do this alone. I required help. I needed strength, and I needed direction. I stood in the moonlight, and said a silent prayer to the heavens, asking for help. I sought guidance to move forward, my cry a simple, uncomplicated request.

Something inside me informed me I had to reflect the same principles the moon used. I had to draw on the strength of another. However, I didn't think I had any fight left in me, the continual battle against my negative emotions, had sucked the life from me. Where would I find the strength to go on?

I stood on the illuminated patio, a broken woman. Tears flowed evenly down my cheeks. My life had been destroyed by something so small it can only be seen under a microscope. Seconds passed. A still calmness descended upon me, a peacefulness which transcended all rationale understanding. Random thoughts trickled into my head like rain drops. They offered assistance, provided direction and brought awareness. Unspoken words revealed themselves to me, like a gift, offered from a higher power. These were not words I would have thought of. Wherever they came from, they inspired me, encouraged me, and for the second time in my life, I grasped I had been given a light to follow, and I knew what I had to do.

I became conscious of the impossibility of being able to fix this situation. I had no skill, but God did. If I was to mentally get through this, it would require His strength, His power, His love and His direction, because I was useless. His light had to be reflected through me, if this situation was going to get any better. I didn't understand how to achieve this. I only knew I needed to let go and try something different. I would not give up on my family, not now. Running away was not the answer. It would not solve anything. In fact, it would destroy everything.

My youngest child lay in that room, tormented. I would not turn my back on him when he needed me the most. And my daughter was yet to be told.

"You can live opposite of what you profess, but you cannot live opposite of what you believe." - Dallas Willard

Chapter 53

Reawakening

"Patience and perseverance have a magical effect, before which difficulties disappear and obstacles vanish."
*- **John Quincy Adams***

My son withdrew for a whole forty-eight hours. For him, this lengthy phase of self-isolation enabled his mind to have a quiet time to process and comprehend the new, unidentified terrain we presented before him. It also provided a moment in time for examination and calculation of all the options. It also offered him a safe haven to restructure a progressive future plan.

To a casual spectator if they viewed this scene, it may have resembled a room filled with serenity and tranquillity. They may have detected a slight level of discord. As his mother, I witnessed the true underlying current that raged and churned within him, as he lay like a statue, face down upon his bed.

During those long forty-eight hours, I was like a ghost, cold, trapped between two worlds, one of self-provocation and one to placate my child. I sat at the side of his bed and gently touched and smoothed his blanket-covered leg. As I sat with him, I questioned what I had done. My behaviour and its consequences had caused so much pain to the people I loved the most. Why didn't I consider that before I shoved a needle in my arm?

Internally, my own personal torrent of rain tried to drench me, soaking me in self-pity and condemnation, but instead of listening to the torment, I focused on transmitting strength and positivity. This action kept me out of the rainstorm that loomed overhead.
An electric shock collided instantly with the negative words that threatened me. This was my son. This was not a time for self-indulgence or self-pity. It was time to really start to practise the reflection tactic I had been shown.

I had to put on my protective rain coat and get out of this entire negative deluge. I knew I had to generate more optimistic thoughts if

I was to positively uphold and endorse a vibrant future for us all. As the time progressed, with my words, I endeavoured to convey a positive outcome to him. I also made a serious effort at being light hearted, but I sometimes struggled with my awful performance. How could I tell my son that everything would be fine, that nothing would change, when in actual fact, I did not know if these words were true?

I found I had to lie, then try and believe in that lie myself. I guess that's what faith is about, believing in something that is not really in front of you, but could potentially be a reality.

The hour glass tilted, little by little, until it finally, totally, fell over. My son released himself from his solitary confinement, ready to once again re-engage with the world. Relief saturated my world, joy flooded me, and my spirits soared. He emerged renewed and ready to fight alongside me.

My earth, my son, once shattered, was now reborn, stronger, firmer and more versatile than before. His internal storm stilled, which enabled his life to restart and move forward. His life returned to the mundane, everyday practices of school, friends and living. This comforted and reassured me of his wellbeing. I watched as my legacy to the world rebuilt his dreams and forged his own precious path into the future.

Time is the best healer. Young people live their lives in perpetual personal expectation and unyielding aspirations, thus, my personal crisis, gladly, became insignificant in his busy world.

If I had the opportunity to pick between extreme happiness and extreme sorrow, I would choose extreme sorrow. For in times of happiness, we tend to forget what really matters in life, and some of us treat life with insufferable arrogance and follow idle pursuits. Yet in times of extreme sorrow, we remember where we have been, who we really are. Our eyes are opened to remember our humble beginnings, and we learn to rely on others. We also learn to trust, and we see God, or what you may call a higher power, sometimes for the very first time.

Chapter 54

The sun lights my world
"How wonderful it is that nobody need wait a single moment before starting to improve the world."
- Anne Frank

I knew that revealing my predicament to my twenty-year-old daughter would be different, but just as hard as it was to tell my son. The situation, language and expressions would need to be adapted to accommodate her personality, as she is nothing like her brother. I didn't expect the same reaction from her. Actually, I was unsure how she would react to the news. She could easily break down in hysterics or simply step over it and not accept it.

My daughter, her warmth blanketed me and penetrated my darkness. She always made me feel important in her life. However, her sincerity and naturalness sometimes overwhelmed me. If I was to be totally removed from her, I would be condemned to eternal night. I could not entertain this thought, as I would never be the same without her by my side.

My first born child, Jade, was born in a harsh and harmful time, trapped in a spiralling rabbit hole of immorality, destruction and depravity. She never asked to be part of my alternate, immoral life, she was there by default, made to endure a life of hardship. If we had anchored in that life, it could have been deadly to both of us.

Thankfully, after six years, I completely disconnected from this port, never to sail into or revisit that harbour again. I chose to shelter and protect her from the harsh reality of the world her father and I shared, and moved her to a different waterfront haven, the Gold Coast.

That night, just a few nights before, on the patio, I was shown to look beyond the obvious and have faith in things unseen. It also instructed me to try and hand my negative feelings, like losing her, out into the universe. They say 90% of what you worry about never comes to fruition, so why waste the effort? However, I found this easier said than done. My efforts to stifle the dark passenger were improving every day, but my progress was sometimes a bit slow. I would win this battle, even if it took me my whole life.

I needed my daughter by my side. I didn't want to do this journey without her. I needed her optimism and her light, as I knew they would carry me through the hard times. I would walk over the burning coals laid out before me, and let the blisters form wherever they may.

"Do not anticipate trouble, or worry about what may never happen. Keep in the sunlight."

- Benjamin Franklin

Chapter 55

A message from a pure heart

"Have courage for the great sorrows of life, and patience for the small ones. And when you have laboriously accomplished your daily task, go to sleep in peace. God is awake."
- Victor Hugo

Another sleepless night faded into the distance, a pattern I hoped would not become habitual. Daybreak dawned, my husband's light, nasal exhalations roused me from my multi-layered, meaningful thoughts. I stirred gently and effortlessly manoeuvred myself from the bed. I found my black bike shorts and a short-sleeved T-shirt and quietly dressed myself. At the back door, waiting for me, were my well-worn favourite running shoes.

I slipped noiselessly out the door to embark on a long, thoughtful run. I needed to clear my head before I meet my daughter. Running was a great distraction for me, and it generally soothed me, especially when I was feeling stressed or upset, both of which I felt this morning.

My feet found an easy rhythm on the hard bitumen surface. I watched as a cloudless, pink day emerged from the deep purple ashes of the night. A spectacular sight. This was my favourite time of day. I ran towards a golden orb, as it rose far out on the horizon. It didn't take long before a beautiful, clear sky surfaced. Even though the morning was still cool, sweat beaded on my forehead and upper lip, it trickled down the base of my spine and was absorbed by my T-Shirt.

I ran my customary six kilometres, my mind much clearer. I was ready to meet my daughter and deliver my news. I hoped I didn't have too many more of these occasions left as I didn't know how many more sleepless nights I could handle.
John and I drove to meet her at the local shopping centre. We had planned to do a bit of shopping and then enjoy a light lunch before heading home.

Our task completed, we stood beside our vehicles. I lifted my face to bathe in the radiance and warmth of the sun's rays whilst Jade chatted happily at my side. I turned to look at her, her face alight with enthusiasm.

She passionately embraced life and loved every aspect of it. Her conversation enlightened me on her new adventures and experiences, which brought pure joy to my heavy heart and a smile to my lips. Communication had never been a problem between us. It would never be an issue for her. Her life was an open book filled with amazement and laughter. Silences are rare in her company. My problem would be getting her full attention.

John distantly sauntered behind us, which offered us both time and space to have a practical talk. I looked deeply, expressively into her immense grey-blue eyes. I delicately and tenderly touched her arm, to obtain her full attention. She suddenly fell silent. She knew I had something important to say. Her eyes flicked back towards John, and then focussed again on me, as she sought reassurance from us that everything was fine.

I spoke truthfully. My words were carefully chosen. I clearly relived the painful details of my youth. I went on to tell her about the consequences of these actions and the consequences and challenges that we faced today. Shock initially coursed through her, visible to any bystander. Tears welled in her eyes, her face turned a pale grey, her legs trembled beneath her, and her voice became unsteady.

She stood silently for a long time, unmoving. After a long moment, she sympathetically and tearfully embraced me, holding me tight against her body. Her tears wet the flimsy shirt which lightly covered my shoulder. I felt her warm breath, as she whispered in my ear, the sweet fragrance of her flavoured chewing gum rose up to touch my nose. A message of hope rung in my ear "it's okay, Mum. Nothing is going to happen to you. I'll pray that you will be healed".

She untangled herself from our embrace, leaving me speechless. I had completed my task, delivered my news. The question was, how would she react once she realised the full extent of the problem we faced?

This beautiful child of mine lived her life in complete optimism and hope. I wished I was more like her. She experienced life fully. She chose to cherish every moment, build happy dreams and lay down joyful memories. Me, I just got the task done, usually as fast as possible. I didn't stop and cherish, or even view, the surrounding scenery. I wondered just how much of life I had already missed because of this. I stupidly drove myself to achieve and achieve. I was stubborn, determined and ambitious. Sad, in reality. She embraced happiness, whereas I embraced success. I think she chose a lot more wisely than I had.

She believed and lived by the fact that hope was a constant fire that burnt in her heart. It was something that didn't go out, even in dark and difficult times, and this situation would be no different. Her hope provided her with optimism and expectation that tomorrow would always be better. She is a strong woman of faith and lived her life according to this conviction. She also believed that her philosophy was to be shared, and everyone else could grasp its concept and embrace it as she did. I loved this innocence in her. I was just thankful she couldn't see into the depths of my soul and see the darkness that sometimes raged within me.

As I recounted and narrated the history of my circumstances to the children, it brought me to the realisation that I needed help emotionally. This was a concept I had never grasped before. My perception was that this was a sign of weakness. Internally, I believed I should be able to deal with my own problems. However, I felt a real, strong need to seek out more personal information regarding my condition, maybe even discuss my feelings with a counsellor. I knew seeing a counsellor meant you had to open up and allow them access to your deeper self. Scary stuff. I also knew they were trained to see beyond what other people didn't, and this frightened me. I feared they would judge me, condemn, reject and criticise me. But, my need to seek help overruled my feelings of fear.

"Faith is all that dreamers need
to see into the future".

- Jim Stovall

Chapter 56

A great support
"One of the most tragic things I know about human nature is that all of us tend to put off living. We are all dreaming of some magical rose garden over the horizon--instead of enjoying the roses that are blooming outside our windows today."
- Dale Carnegie

I stumbled across an organisation called the Hepatitis Council. This organisation specialised in assisting people and their family members in the same situation as me. I wondered why no one had referred me to them before. Even in all the folders that contained my research, I didn't locate them. I couldn't understand why I hadn't heard of them, or why the GP hadn't referred me to them. I looked through all my research and found it predominantly included scientific literature, which is what I was seeking at the time.

After a few days, and much internal debate, I summoned the courage to telephone the service for support and to substantiate my findings. Questions raced through my mind, as I hastily dialled the eight digit number. I pondered how I would begin this conversation. What would I say? Could I really disclose my sordid tale to an absolute stranger? Would they judge and ridicule me? I would soon know the answers. I couldn't stop the rising feelings of anxiety and apprehension, as they had become my silent companions.

Our telephone lines connected. A persistent ring bellowed in my ear. Internal, whispered words tried to coerce me to disregard the call, they stated the whole prospect of seeking help from unknown people was unnecessary, and I didn't need to go through this. What could they offer me that I could not do myself? I refused to allow their words to prevent me from seeking what I needed: help and support.

My thoughts were interrupted by a pleasant female voice. She inquired about my needs. For a moment I couldn't speak. I was dumbfounded, amazed I had actually done it. I had never sought support like this before. I was breaking new ground in the Laurie category! My pride was thrown out the window, overtaken by a basic human need. The drawn-out silence between us prompted me to speak. Embarrassed at my slow reaction, I stumbled over my words like a child learning to walk. The softly spoken woman intently listened and was able to decipher the meaning behind my jumbled words. She must have been very intuitive, because I doubted even I would be able to discern the message or even the language I spoke. Thankfully, she could, and I was forwarded to a professional counsellor.

My fears were promptly and completely washed away as soon as the man spoke. His sensitive concern shrouded me, bringing peace to my troubled world. He genuinely cared. I heard it in his voice. His words more than just reassured and eased my worries; they completely banished my previously held doubts.

The competence and composure of the individuals I dealt with at the Hepatitis Council was exceptional. My conversation ended, and I felt entirely at ease. I knew I now had a fighting chance at survival. Even though I had mountains of research, stating facts on survival rates and disease progression, I still didn't believe it was relevant in my case, until I actually heard it spoken directly to me from this man. Speaking to this counsellor transformed me. I noticed that the old, spirited character I knew before this saga began started to resurface. After my positive experience with the Council, I advocated and recommended the benefits of a visit to both my son and husband. Both of them went into Brisbane and had a personal face to face visit with the same counsellor.

A noticeable, constructive change occurred after their visit. I knew it had something to do with the empowerment and support that was tendered to each of us by the Hepatitis Council. I never inquired about my boy's meeting, as I felt it was a very private occasion, and one I did not feel privy to. I do know the Hepatitis Council had a very positive impact on all of us though, and I was so grateful for the input they had.

> *"Kind words can be short, and easy to speak,
> but their echoes, are truly endless."*
> *- Mother Teresa*

Chapter 57

Reflection on life

As an adult writing this story, it is easy to look back and reflect to see that I wasted so much of my life and my energy protecting myself. My isolation from the world prevented me from creating real, sustainable relationships. It was a form of self-imprisonment. I was too scared to actually live and engage outside of the comfort and familiarity of the security of my castle. For a long time, I wasn't consciously aware of what I was doing.

Living a life dominated by fear such as this, is not genuinely living; it is, in fact, just existing. My life was bound by anguish and doubt. In essence, I felt like it was a desolate, lonely highway in an overcrowded city. I lived amongst many people, but I was a total stranger who wore a mask, moulded to what I perceived to be the needs of others. I would only remove my mask in the confines and safety of my castle. Those closest to me, a select few, were able to see what genuinely lay beneath.

I found that you can dwell with many, but still your silent cries, the cries of the heart, are not heard, simply because you refuse to let them be heard. When I finally dared to release myself from my self-imposed prison, I somehow became more aligned with my inner self, and glimpsed a sight of who I could be. I slowly learnt to trust people and built some meaningful relationships. Like my daughter, I experienced moments of pure joy. I also learnt to laugh for the first time with real meaning, something you can't do on your own.

Learning to live unencumbered by my self-doubts, blessed me with moments of peace in the midst of all of this turmoil. Over time, I learnt that positive, strong roots could grow stronger in my life if I watered and tended to them. My life transformed when I adopted this new found philosophy. I was not always brilliant at applying it, but when I did, I was like a climbing rose, bound tightly on a supporting trellis. I gained strength, support and love, as well as the ability to share my pain and sorrow.

Chapter 58

Our education is never over
"Do not go where the path may lead, go instead where there is no path and leave a trail."
- Ralph Waldo Emerson

I allowed Hepatitis C to initially steal my life, but it also gave me something in return. It gave me much more than it took from me. It opened my eyes to a world I never imagined was possible with John. John became my best friend. We shared a single purpose and a common goal. A true and deep bond formed between us. We shared the same song, and when I forgot the words, he could recite them back to me to keep me going.

He became the turret in my castle wall. He protected me and nurtured my wounded spirit. He held me in the palm of his hand, provided support and encouragement, as well as assisted my actions towards treatment. He was able to capture and sift through the good and bad in our lives, stack and store everything worth keeping, and throw the rest away, discarding it like garbage.

Our lives became like a powerful symphony, days filled with high notes followed by crashing crescendos. I was up and down, believing, unbelieving, suffering, enduring, yet, John persisted through all my emotions, a sky ablaze with dazzling colour, a truly magical occurrence. I witnessed the whole spectrum of emotions while I waited for the specialist's appointment and John stood firm beside me. He fixed my brokenness and pulled me out of the pit when I fell in and placed my feet back on solid ground.

Together we created strategies to positively move forward and with his help I was able to fully accept my situation. I had found an appreciation and respect for the journey I was on. I came to realise it held some purpose. I may never understand this purpose, but I knew a life's lesson would be learnt. My education and teachers changed daily. At the rate I was going, I thought I was being fast tracked to university.

Life became my priority. My diagnosis brought me face to face with my own mortality and I discovered a new found passion for the journey I embarked on. I planted tiny seeds of hope, which slowly grew and strengthened over time. I also had a new found respect for my own human fragility. Every moment in my life became more meaningful than the last. Each moment was to be enjoyed, not ignored. I had overlooked many meaningful connections in my life and I would not do this anymore.

I had a sudden realization that there were many concealed, unknown mysteries that surrounded my life. Life and all the promises it held used to pass me by unnoticed. I now allowed it to linger so I could explore it. Some situations and experiences had already been lost forever, buried in the annals of time, never to be unearthed. These were missed lessons in life which would never be explained to me, and they represented missed opportunities to learn something important. Lessons I would never learn under those conditions again, and experiences I would never get to enjoy, because I filled my life with trivial, insignificant affairs, instead of stopping and smelling the roses. This was a phrase often thrown at me, from many different angles, and one I truly didn't understand or appreciate until I was struck by a sledgehammer. The strike so intense it made me stop and assess everything.

I was grateful for that jolt, it was a wakeup call. I can honestly say it changed everything about me. Not overnight, sometimes the changes were subtle as I crawled and sometimes the changes were dramatic as I leapt forward. But, I woke up each day with a new vigour, a new zest, for the day. I was more thankful for every day and every moment. Things that once bothered me didn't anymore.
I found a sense of peace. I believed God placed His hand upon my life and breathed life into what was once a decaying corpse. I found and held onto a belief and conviction: I was going to beat HCV.

"It's not what you look at that matters, it's what you see."

- Henry David Thoreau

Chapter 59

Life in its reality
"It is easier to go down a hill than up, but the view is from the top."
- Arnold Bennett

Once my eyes were fully opened, I spent a lot of time reflecting on my attitude, behaviours and actions, and I was shown things I didn't want to see. My mirror image was not the same image as the one I imagined. I came to realise, I hadn't invested my time wisely. I was self-centred, insensitive, complicated, sometimes spiteful as well as being ruthless, forbidding and unkind to those I loved, and others.

I asked myself reflective questions including, "If I stood in a court room right now, this very moment, and sat in the witness box before my God, my maker, being questioned about my life, what would be my excuses for all the people I have hurt, and the carnage my actions and my words have caused?" What would I say in my defense? Did I really appreciate the days I was given? Did I take things for granted? Did I appreciate the things others did for me? Did I help others, or was I selfish and self-centred? The answers that came to me were not good. I knew I had a lot to be accountable for.

The soft, fluffy wool had definitely been removed from my eyes. I accurately saw who I was, and I didn't like the person I saw. I observed, firsthand, the devastating effects my harsh words and actions caused others. I couldn't take any of it back, but I could use the time I had left to change and make amends. I vowed to change my behaviour and change fast.

"The heart of the problem is a problem with the heart. You're just a prayer away from a change of heart. Finding relief in your problem is fine, but it will not cure the problem."
"My environment can give me relief from sin and tension, only the Lord can cure it."

Dr. Henry Brandt

Chapter 60

Growing in spirit
"Problems may only be avoided by exercising good judgment. Good judgment may only be gained by experiencing life's problems."
- Jim Stovall

Changes don't happen quickly, but they do happen when you persevere, which is what I chose to do. Books by Norman Vincent Peale, Anthony Robbins, Florence Littauer and Steven Covey dominated my study and replaced my once loved Stephen King and Dean Koontz. Like a ravenous lioness, I devoured and analysed every word from these brilliant motivational and relationship books, with the desperate plea to positively influence and transform my life.

I aspired to live a better, healthier, more wholesome life. To effectively do this, I needed to put into practice the teaching of my new mentors. This required a whole new outlook, a transformation of my behaviours, my interactions with others, my speech and my thought processes. It was tough, as it challenged my preconceived concepts and ideals.

I visualized myself as a spectator at my own funeral. People milled around as they drank steamy hot cups of coffee and ate moist, freshly baked cakes. They discussed my life as they witnessed it. Who would be there? How had I impacted their life? What would they say about me? What sort of person did they perceive me to be? What stories would they remember? Would the stories possess a positive or negative undertone? Visualising this scenario made me realise, I did not want to leave a legacy that reflected unconstructive, hurtful or critical events. Rather, I wanted people to reflect upon me as a worthy, compassionate and helpful person.

My new mentors openly discussed the importance of learning to trust, as well as demonstrating traits such as reliability, integrity, ability and strength. Another key factor included the ability to expose your vulnerabilities and seek support. Well, that was a hard one for me. My internal radar didn't like this task. To me, trust was earned by actions, not words. Trusting others required that I let my guard down, and most of my earlier experiences of this had a negative feel to them. However, these books informed me my perception was based upon my experiences and was therefore distorted. It was simply a symbol of my own projected guilt and fears. Their words made me reflect more deeply, and I reconsidered my values and beliefs yet again.

I recalled the day when John and I had an in-depth conversation by the pool. I had completely exposed myself and my vulnerabilities to him and he stood by me. Actually, he rose to the challenge and fought repeatedly to keep me on solid ground. So, my mentors' philosophy did work; I had witnessed it. I recalled another event twenty years ago when John had not judged or condemned me for the behaviours of my past. I realised trust doesn't mean that the person has to be perfect, just that they do their best in the situation they are in at the time, and John had proven this to me time and time again.

The question was whether or not I could trust others outside of my circle. Did I dare to try it? I decided to proceed, regardless of any perceived difficulties. I would not allow my subconscious to ruin my life, or cause me to live a life a fear, any longer. I had proven the models taught in these books could work. I had witnessed the benefits, by testing my husband. I would not be denied the fruit this lesson held. I would test it on another source. I would try their principles again, on my friends.

> *"Life is either a daring adventure or nothing. Security does not exist in nature, nor do the children of men as a whole experience it. Avoiding danger is no safer in the long run than exposure."*
>
> *- Hellen Keller*

Chapter 61

Perceptions, are they really real?

"The ultimate measure of a man is not where he stands in moments of comfort and convenience, but where he stands at times of challenge and controversy."
- *Martin Luther King, Jr.*

John and I lived a quiet life. We shared it with only a handful of what we considered to be real friends. We both disliked superficiality, or unnecessary burdens, so we kept our social circle small and discrete. We were private people who disliked living our lives within a public arena, opting for a more clandestine, behind the scenes, approach.

Disclosing my disease outside my immediate family generated a lot of unease for both of us. The stigma associated with HCV, and how it would be perceived, was our primary concern. We both wondered if we would have any friends left, once they knew I was a previous drug user, and had contracted HCV. HCV had the same stigma that HIV did back in the '80s when people were uninformed, ignorant and frightened. They were panicked about infected children in child care facilities, forcing them to be removed. Ridiculous, but true!

Now you may understand some of my concerns for not disclosing my health status to anyone, but I also had the problem of working in a Correctional Facility, where the stigma and discrimination was common and widespread. Hepatitis was a dirty word in prison, and I would never dare to speak about my condition to anyone inside. I thought discrimination and intolerance would have been my punishment. I didn't need or want any more of that; I carried my own reprimand with me everywhere.

It is a very personal decision to disclose, and by law, you don't have to. There are a few exceptions, but in general you don't have to inform anyone.

Once again, I would refer you to the Hepatitis Council, as they will support and encourage you, as well as provide you with all the information you need to manage your life with HCV. Words cannot describe just how much they helped me. I will be eternally grateful to them for that.

"It is time for us to stand and cheer for the doer, the achiever, the one who recognizes the challenge and does something about it."

Vince Lombardi

Chapter 62

Inner demons are not what they seem

"Look not mournfully into the past. It comes not back again. Wisely improve the present. It is thine. Go forth to meet the shadowy future, without fear."
- Henry Wadsworth Longfellow

I was ready. I knew it was time to reach out to my friends. I had been hedging phones calls for too long, unable to deal with the situation, but I felt stronger and equipped with enough knowledge to answer questions. Never the less, I was still nervous about their perceptions and reactions.

My new found resolve, assisted by Mr Peale, enabled me to set up my first meeting with my friend, a nurse. I manoeuvred the car into the parking area and sat quietly as I tried to settle my stomach and prepare my speech. All around me, diligent people with laughing, noisy children pushed food-laden trolleys. I got out of the car and slowly walked towards the heavy plate glass automated doors. I saw her as she stood observing the chaos and commotion of the busy centre.

We had met each other eight years earlier, when I became the manager of the gymnasium she worked in. I initially found her blunt, challenging and discontented with the world and her life, and I liked her straight away. There was something about her that drew me to her immediately. I think she reminded me a bit of myself. Together, over the years, a strong friendship grew. We shared plans, ideas, as well as many unfulfilled dreams.

As I walked into the mall, our eyes met. She knew I had something important to discuss. She wasted no time in directing us to the coffee shop and ordered our coffees. After placing the order she turned to face me. Bluntly, she said "what's this all about?" Before I could respond, my eyes filled and overflowed unexpectedly. She touched my arm and guided me to a table for some privacy.

I stared at her and immediately I knew our longstanding friendship would out last turmoils such as this. I probed why I had painstakingly doubted her ability to understand my predicament. She was, after all, a nurse and a great friend. I knew our relationship had been built on mutual trust, respect and support, so why did I doubt it? When I saw her, I knew I could tell her anything. She would accept it, understand and still appreciate what we had.

For the next few minutes, she listened intently as I summarized my plight. I revealed everything. Neither of us touched our coffees whilst I spoke. She stared deeply into my eyes as she processed the information I had given her. A smile danced at the corner of her mouth, she reached for her cup, took a long sip from her now luke warm coffee, and said "is that it? Is that why you have been dismissing my calls? Why didn't you just tell me?"

Over our mugs of delicious coffee, we informally explored every option imaginable. The sweet taste of sugar lingered in my mouth as our conversation drew to a close. We stood and faced each other as we searched for the right words. She grabbed and secured my hand with both of hers and said "HCV doesn't change anything. If anything, it will make you stronger. You will just battle this like everything else in your life. You are a fighter, and don't ever forget it!"

We said our goodbyes, and I carelessly drifted towards the door. That was easier than I thought. Would the others be that simple? I certainly hoped so. Her positive and supportive reaction gave me the fundamental strength and resilience to run the gauntlet and overcome all the self-placed obstacles that had prevented me from getting to this moment.

I was ready and willing to now run that extra mile. I would tell my other close friends today, if possible. I had painstakingly fought and finally silenced my long suffering, tormenting demons, the ones that tried to keep me isolated and alone.

The task set before me was no longer arduous, the mountainous, rocky, inhospitable terrain now distant, replaced by a pleasant welcoming trail. I told my two other closest friends, and I was met by warm-hearted, affectionate people who offered small yet precise waves of hope, love and support. I acknowledged that the tormenting devils in our lives are never quite what we expect, especially when they are met face to face and brought out of the darkness into the light. Identifying this made me admit, I should never have segregated myself from my friends or family. These people wanted to be a part of my life. I stupidly excluded them.

Self-protection, previously, was the foundation of every choice I made. I saw the world differently now. The world I had created was unhealthy and unproductive. My convictions had battered my life. They had destabilized the fragile essence of it, but I had been shown another way. People do care.

My support team had considerably grown in size from two to eight. This new team overtly turned the wheels of life for me, especially when the darkness prevailed. Their presence was a soft breeze, tender, yet compelling. They brought reassurance and comfort to my unstable world. They boosted my hope and encouraged a release from my personalized self-judgment.

I was greatly honoured and deeply touched when they pioneered the new HCV research centre in my living room. I found myself inundated and saturated with referrals to naturopaths, acupuncturists, Chinese nutritionists and doctors. Literature and research papers now camouflaged and concealed the exquisite dappled grey slate, which served as my flooring. Piles of paper not only sprawled out, littering the floor, but clawed and clambered up the walls.

It was exceptional and phenomenal; something I will never forget. The problem was, I had to read it all, then deliberate and debate it with my new learned colleagues. My idle doomsday speculations were totally proven to be unfounded. What I uncovered was gladiators who fought gallantly for my survival. These were professional people who bound themselves body and soul to me, swearing an oath "to endure through this hardship." They became a cohesive group united by courage, confidence and a common goal: my survival.

Chapter 63

A conscious awakening

"God will one day hold us each accountable for all the things He created for us to enjoy, but we refused to do so."
-Rabbanic Saying

Living with HCV challenged me on so many levels. It fractured me on every level, physically, spiritually and emotionally, but it also brought a deep awakening into my life. It brought major changes. It prompted me to review everything I believed in. It prompted me to trust in people again. It increased my level of faith, not only in God, but in humanity. It also prompted me to look at me, and who I had actually become.

I believe life offers all of us choices. Our life experiences can either be negative baggage that we choose to carry around with us, or we can learn to let them go and forgive the people involved. I chose to forgive my parents for what I perceived to be their transgressions, simply because I just didn't want to be one of those people who chose to be hurt 24/7. I wanted them in my life and I certainly needed their support to go forward into the next phase of my life. It was time to put them in the picture.

I sought to craft the right scene. My historical masterpiece simply couldn't be postponed anymore. My family, my father, my mother and my brother, would be told, and I was scared. Our histories had been filled with great pain, and I was unsure of placing my hand on the hot stove again, but I would trust in their commitment and dedication to our new relationship.

My unique family consists of my proud, untamed father. He is an impressive, powerful man, noble and imposing in character and commanding in stature. My territorial and solitary mother is resourceful and adaptable, with feline elegance and stealth, and, lastly, my intelligent, efficient brother, an alert, loyal companion with extremely sharp, quick wit and very agile in temperament. My relationship with each varied considerably and had changed dramatically over time. As my life's situation changed and I grew in wisdom, so did my relationships with each member of my family.

Chapter 64

A true portrait

"What are your choices? Whom are your choices for? Not just for yourself. Chose now whom you will serve, and that choice is going to affect the next generation, and the next generation, and the next. Choice never affects just one person alone. It goes on and on and the effect goes out into geography and history. You are part of history and your choices become part of history."
-Edith Schaeffer

My brother, seven years my junior, was married and a parent himself. He unfortunately was a stranger in my life. My period of earlier forced and then chosen exile from the family prevented me from constructing any strong bonds with my kin. We were two transient bystanders, from the same origin, but our single path had been forcibly divided, and we were sent in opposite directions. By the time I was prepared and equipped to reawaken my relationship with him, it was too late. We were so different, our experiences altered us, and I found no solid ground to rebuild our relationship upon.

Life had tragically torn us apart. I loved him deeply, as the tie between brother and sister is, but we knew absolutely nothing about each other. We were two grown adults unable to recognize the true value and joy that could have developed between us, because it was stolen from us over twenty years ago. A deep, meaningful connection forever lost in the lines on our faces. Instead, the chambers of our hearts held distance, tolerance, patience and charity, whereas laughter, elation, tenderness and expectations should have pumped through every muscle of our beings.

We had a lost attachment, like a stroke that paralyses the body. We needed assistance to regenerate our bond. Maybe this would reunite us. A shared quest to fight a common enemy. Only time would tell.

Despite our lost connection, he was someone I could rely on, a pillar of strength in times of trouble. Telling him would be easier than the other members of my family. The unfortunate part in this scenario was both he and my mother lived over 600km away. I would have to modify my approach and gauge their reactions via a telephone conversation.

I was not nervous as I called his number, as I knew he would be rational and logical with the news. I announced my situation with as much factual information as I had. I kept the sordid tale as brief and concise as possible. Thankfully, with my well-organized, disciplined troops' support, I had all the answers I needed to respond to the many questions he asked. His response was objective and impartial, just as I expected. Two weeks later I received a parcel from him filled with information and expressions of hope and love.

My mother was next to be told. If worrying was an Olympic sport, my mother's living room would be filled with gold medals. I believe she could represent Australia in the London 2012 Olympics. Knowing this about her triggered apprehension in me. I didn't know how to tell her without causing her undue anxiety and panic. I knew I would have to talk to her calmly and candidly. I hoped I could deliver the facts quick enough, before she would gather too many pieces of hardwood and sprint off to construct a bridge we may never cross.

I lifted the phone and dialled her number. I took a big deep breath to flood my body with cool, clean air, to settle my agitated stomach. My warm-up preparations were interrupted by her deep, raspy voice, which disconnected me from my verbal rehearsal. I bared my soul to her. A tiny bird, her chick, with a big song to sing.

The news obviously shocked and stunned her, as a quiet stillness crossed the airways. The coolness of a black night fell upon her warm summer's day. I could hear her subtle sobs, and I knew that tears flowed down her cheeks, even though I couldn't see them. She absorbed every piercing arrow, even though they initiated more suffering and painful injury to her heart.

Delivering this message in this manner was tough. The phone is generally not the best way to clearly enlighten someone of a situation like this. It was, for me, virtually impossible to appropriately impart a message like that using a telephone. I knew the manner it was delivered could misinterpret the message. My tone of voice, as well as the words I used, could change how she comprehended the information. But it was my only option at that time.

I didn't want to cause her undue stress and place another medal on her wall. We ended our conversation with the promise to cherish the gifts each day brought, and not to dwell too much on the destructive forces that may rattle the doors of our lives. I was quite relieved when this conversation was over.

Lastly, I had to tell my father, the commander of the family. He held a very negative view of the medical profession. So my approach needed to be strategically planned and implemented, so I would not receive a lecture on doctor's failures or misdiagnoses.

A timely event arose: his 65th birthday. We planned to celebrate this special occasion as a family event on the Gold Coast. I just had to find the right opportunity to be alone with him. As fortune would have it, he wanted to come for a walk with me along the beach the next morning. I knew this was the moment of truth.

I awoke to a cold, dark winter's morning. The red fluorescent numbers on the old motel digital clock advised me it was 5:55am. It was time for my true life portrait to be unveiled. Feelings of uneasiness and restlessness washed over me, as I pulled on my warm gym clothes and my favourite comfortable running shoes. I kissed John goodbye and set off to embark on the last leg of my journey before the next chapter began.

The day had just begun. A ball of flames rose out of the earth, encased in a brilliant, deep-red, fiery halo. It floated carelessly on the horizon. A natural wonder which brought a fresh start, and hope, in a world full of chaos. The wind battered my face. Grains of airborne sand struck me from every angle. My hair struggled under its elastic constraint and thrashed frenziedly. It obstructed my view and annoyed me. A couple of fearless surfers in black, full piece wetsuits braved the cold water and paddled out into the winter swells. Only a few valiant walkers shared the concrete walkway with us, which enabled us to talk freely and openly.

We started our discussion with the usual topics of politics and the family, but mainly, we just wanted to enjoy the moment and each other's company. Finally, there was a break in the conversation, and I jumped in and divulged the details of my story to him.
He didn't understand everything I told him, but he understood enough. I spent the next hour sharing all I had learnt over the last few months.

As we rounded an unfamiliar bend in the walkway, I was touched by a bright yellow beam of light. Sunlight struck my uncovered eyes, and alerted me to our location. Unknowingly, we walked right past our hotel. Dad voicelessly walked beside me, entrenched in profound thought, clearly troubled by the newly presented problem I had placed before him.

I broke the lingering silence by revealing our location and informing him that without realizing it, we had both walked beyond our hotel. Laughter fractured the tension between us. We turned around and leisurely strolled back to our beachside hotel and our comfortable chic rooms.

As we neared the hotel, he finally spoke. He was interested in my intentions. He wanted to know how I was going to deal with the situation and what plans I had made. I informed him of my appointment with the gastroenterologist and of my plans to consult my naturopath. He was content with these calculated future plans. However, he wanted to also assist me with research and access another naturopath's opinion on my behalf.

The task was done. It had been easier than I thought. All my preconceived notions were once again unfounded. I had been accepted by everyone, not rejected and shunned as I thought I would be.

The rest of our weekend passed without incident. No-one discussed my infection, and dad and I didn't speak about the content of our previous beachside conversation. The rest of his birthday was celebrated in a stylish and cheerful style, then we all parted again to our own lives.

Chapter 65

Fears are not always founded
"The only good is knowledge, and the only evil is ignorance."
Diogenes Laertius

My entire immediate family now understood the perils that John and I faced. We had one last quest to complete; John's family needed to be put into the picture. Our connection with them had been quite strained over the years. Expectations not met, perceptions misunderstood and lots of communication problems. All of us were responsible for the lost connection between us. Unfortunately, a detachment had formed between us, caused by distance, time constraints and personality differences, which led to limited and sporadic association.

I believed the prospect of telling his mother our story humiliated him. I also thought this information may potentially ruin any future relationships between us. His mother had never approved of our union and this had significantly contributed to the problems between us. Over the years, I withheld my own unvoiced feelings of rejection from her and the rest of the family. All of this influenced John's and my perception of a negative reaction to our news, and this made both of us very nervous.

We wanted to convey our message to her directly, so we could answer her questions and offer her a comprehensive explanation if she asked for one. So, we invited her to our place for the weekend. Four months had passed since my diagnosis, and both of us were very familiar, comfortable even, with our situation. However, we were still reluctant and scared to tell her.

After she arrived and settled into her assigned room, we enjoyed a delightful and tasty dinner, followed by cold drinks on the patio. We shared glasses of chilled beverages and inconspicuous, ordinary conversation. I could see both John and his mother were relaxed and at ease with each other. A pleasant peace and understanding passed between them, an alcohol-enriched view of the world and life.

It was time for me to leave and allow them some private time to talk. I subtly and tenderly squeezed my husband's shoulder and gave him a reassuring look of support and encouragement. I excused myself from their company and carelessly wandered into our generously-proportioned, brick and wood kitchen to wash the dinner dishes, which were casually stacked in the double stainless steel sink. I didn't hear any of the spoken words.

The kitchen clean and tidy, I felt it was time to rejoin the conversation and offer support, as well as provide information, if it was needed.

My mother-in-law sat quietly in the dark, staring deep into the moonlit night. Light danced and bounced on the surface of the pool and the stars twinkled high in the sky. Confused tears plunged down her cheeks. Her eyes searched mine. She reached for answers to the questions she would never ask. She simply told me she was sorry. This memory will be forever etched in my memory, because it was then that I realised she genuinely did care what happened to me. That night, we held no schedule. I spoke late into the night revealing the mysteries of HCV and everything I knew about my condition. I believe she left our house with sufficient information to understand our situation, our intentions, as well as her own personal risk factors. After she left our house, a sense of relief and amazement flowed over us. The task was finally complete. We could now enter the next phase of this journey, to meet the specialist and all the surprises that would hold.

Telling the family was easier than we thought. Harrowing, yet more positive than we both ever imagined. However, it also came with a deep sense of regret. Feelings of disappointment fuelled our fires of remorse, as we comprehended our shortcomings of not being able to inform them earlier, or including them in the initial phase of this journey.

"Be not angry that you cannot make others as you wish them to be, since you cannot make yourself as you wish to be."

- Thomas A. Kempis

Chapter 66

Exposing HCV.
"Make your own recovery the first priority in your life.
- Robin Norwood

I love the words of that song, "time keeps on slipping, slipping, slipping into the future," because it's exactly true. You can't touch it or place it in a box. All any of us can do is leave a mark where we have been. Time doesn't care about your concerns or what's happening in the world. It has a job to do and it does it faithfully.

As the specialist appointment loomed, drawing nearer each day, I felt more and more like a passenger on board a unique ship. A ship which had undertaken an essential course, and its destination was completely unknown to me.

One day the wait was over. I would finally meet the man. This was the day I had been waiting for. I was ready, but also sincerely uneasy. I woke early to the sun as it deviously peered through the wooden blinds above my head. Deep, rhythmic breathing harmonized with the noises of the early dawn. Quietly, I lay and rehearsed the words I wanted to say. In my mind I systematically went over everything I had previously learnt. Sleep was impossible. My mind raced with possible scenarios and intangible outcomes. My husband lay serene and peaceful beside me, his back turned towards me.

I deliberately tried not to disturb his sleeping mass as I checked the time. 5am. It was hours before my historic trip. I knew a run would settle my nerves, so I unhurriedly slipped out of bed, picked up my clothes, strewn on the floor, and dressed quietly in the lounge room. I chose a long, slow 8km route, as I knew I needed time to think. My MP3 player's earphones settled snugly in my ears. Techno and hip hop tunes synchronized my stride and carried me safely on my journey.

An hour later, I returned, hot and sweaty, to the pleasant aroma of coffee. John stood in the kitchen annoying fragrant meat as it sizzled in a fry pan, bacon. Hmm, I loved bacon, but I didn't think it would be possible for me to eat anything, as my stomach churned with nerves. A simple coffee and shower would be all the sustenance I would be able to partake of this morning. The hours passed slowly. My world became the sands that filled the hour glass, and every grain fell slowly, which was an anxious taunt.

The hour glass finally emptied and I knew I was about to enter into the next phase of the Hep C journey. My questions would be answered and I would be able to see the ultimate destination of the ship I was a passenger on.

Over the last few months, John and I had many long, silent, reflective drives, and this one was no exception. As I closed my eyes, I could hear the rhythmical hum of the car's engine. I tried to focus on its tempo to calm my endless theories. What I really wanted to do was formulate a plan.

We arrived after an hour's silent drive. I walked up the stairs to the waiting room, checked in and was ready for my appointment. The staff were discrete, friendly and welcoming. I noticed the room was light and airy, filled with various faceless people as they sat and read magazines.

I joined John by the water chiller and chose a magazine. In spite of this, I found it impossible to focus my mind on it. The words were all muddled, the sentences unreadable and faceless pictures adorned every page. My body was wound up like a tightly coiled spring. If I was released now, I thought I would spin for at least an hour.

This was an interval I didn't really want. It required all my strength to sit and wait as my body demanded to stand and pace. A familiar and warm hand engulfed mine. It brought forth a slight sense of peace, taking the edge off my inner turmoil. John gazed affectionately at me and said, "no matter what happens, I will always love you."

I leant over and rested my head on his broad, heavily burdened shoulder. Right then, I recognised that my world was a much happier place when I had someone to share it with. I still found it hard to believe he was still with me. For better or for worse, in sickness and in health, these vows were in fact a reality. I realised worry and suffering were self-indulgent and self-imposed, but to understand the real value of happiness, you have to have a true connection with another human being, and I did, this great humble presence beside me.

A sturdy, robust man wearing hospital scrubs suddenly appeared. He stood and searched the many faces in the room. His booming voice resonated in my ears. My name rang out, and his eyes fell on me as I promptly stood up. He sauntered down the narrow, carpeted corridor, then stopped and rested outside the entrance to an office. I presumed it was his treatment room. He waited patiently for our arrival. His big, outstretched hand greeted us, then he introduced himself and ushered us into his office. His smiling face, complete with spectacles, did not display any of the weariness he must have felt from his pre-dawn surgery schedule.

The conversation commenced. He was candid, considerate and spoke with sensitivity. He explained my test results and the forthcoming potential scenarios and options. He dropped a bombshell on me when he informed me I might not actually be infected. The previous test had just detected the fact I had come in contact with the disease, but 20% of people automatically defeat the virus themselves, and the rest go on to have what is called chronic infection. I was stunned to learn this fact.

All the months of lost sleep, agonizing over my future were pointless. Although, a voice inside me told me I would be infected. I simple wasn't that lucky. So he wrote me another pathology request, this time for more in-depth tests such as a PCR Qualitative (to make sure I had a live virus) and Quantitative (how much of the virus was in my blood) as well as a genotype and liver function tests. My genotype test was important, as specific genotypes respond better to treatment and the results also determine the length of time a person is on treatment, if I was able to access it. I wished for Genotype two or three as I would only require twenty four weeks of treatment and it was a lot easier to cure. Genotype one was the hardest to cure and required forty-eight weeks of treatment. With my luck, I would most likely have Genotype one.

I was relieved I had spent so much time and effort researching, as I could understand the facts as he presented them to us. How daunting this scenario must be if a person has no prior knowledge of this disease. As I sat and listened to him unravel the secrets HCV held, it became apparent that this disease was not widely discussed, or understood. I was amazed to find out that 130-170 million people throughout the world suffered with a form of Hepatitis. What unsettled me most was the fact that 350,000 people die each year from its affects. These figures blew my mind, but they also frightened me. I knew I was not alone, but, that is a lot of people! I also came to realise that your average, well-intentioned doctor doesn't usually deal with infectious diseases like this, so their knowledge can be limited. It is a complex disease, which the public doesn't really understand. I know I didn't.

Our discussion continued. We covered treatment options, liver care and disease management. He also explained I needed to have the results of the other tests and a liver biopsy done before we could proceed any further. The thought of both terrified me. I could not imagine being fully awake whilst a long thin tube, resembling a barbecue skewer, punctured the upper right side of my body, then was wedged about half way inside me to take a cross section of liver cells. Our meeting concluded on this note and an appointment was made for my liver biopsy.

The perception I held in my mind of the liver biopsy procedure really terrified me. I tried to keep my fears to myself, but daily, I longed for a life without these difficulties. I knew I needed to gain strength and courage to look fear in the face and conquer it. I had to do what I thought I couldn't do. I had to find and hold onto a sense of peace to get me through what lay ahead.

On my dark days, my friends would constantly remind me that the best diamonds were made under extraordinary pressure. Well, I thought I would be brilliant at the end of this, if that was the truth. I completed all the blood tests, the ultrasound and the liver biopsy, and none of them were as bad as the scenarios that were created in my mind.

Chapter 67

A door slams shut
> *"As strong as my legs are, it is my mind that has made me a champion."*
> **-Michael Johnson**

In due course, all the results returned and an appointment was scheduled for me to return to the specialist. There was no turning back now. My journey was about to really begin; a poignant moment which would define my life. The door to my life of forty-two years slammed shut, nice and tight, behind me. It would never be able to be opened ever again.

Death was not my biggest fear. Taking the risk to really live and see this through to the end, was. Whatever was said today would determine the course my life would take. My irritated, unfilled stomach grumbled with pangs of anxiety, not because I felt hungry, but because I was concerned about what was about to happen. Here, I sat in the same waiting room, with the same physical feelings coursing through my body. I was a little more anxious this time than the last time, most likely because I knew more was at stake.

I tried to fill the void in time by flicking through countless, meaningless magazines. My fingers quickly turned pages without considering any of the actual content. I felt compelled to sit silently, but internally, I felt like I was on speed. My inner furnace was stoked. Sweat beaded on my upper lip, and at the same time, dripped down the small of my back. All my neurons fired simultaneously, cells collided. A leg twitch formed and caused twinges of pain to dance down to my ankle.

I looked up and there he stood. He beckoned us into his room, it felt like Ground Hog Day. Here, the truth would be revealed. I felt panic rise up in me. I wanted to run. Did I really want the answers? Was it better to know, or not to know? Any second now, I would have to make a decision. There was an awkward moment before my body engaged in movement.

A reflection of my first experience on a rollercoaster struck me. I remembered sitting in a carriage, fully restrained, as it slowly crept towards an unbelievable height. For a split second, from this height, I could see the big picture for what it truly was, and then I started the fast descent. My mind wanted only to scream whilst my hands, like eagle's talons, firmly gripped the safety bar in front of me. I thought I was prepared for this moment, but I wasn't ready to hear what was about to be said. I wasn't ready to partake of the penalty I knew was going to be imposed today.

Nothing could prepare me for the twists and turns I was about to experience. In a matter of moments, I would know how bad my liver damage was. I would learn how much virus was coursing through my veins, and the big question may well be answered. Was I going to die from it? I didn't really want it answered, but I knew I would ask it anyway.

John and I both walked into his homey office. He greeted us with his mischievous and lively manner, shook our hands at the door as was his customary fashion, and ushered us to our seats. He walked behind his large, messy desk and positioned himself comfortably in his chair. His unwavering gaze informed me that he was about to tell me something very serious, and that I needed to be ready.

His matter-of-fact, approachable attitude was what I liked most about him. He explained the biopsy results showed I had cirrhosis and a lot of inflammation around my liver. My mind began to recall some research I had conducted on this topic. This was not a good start.

He then succinctly spoke directly to my partner. He explained I needed to access treatment straight away. Time was of the essence. The state of my disease, at that point, could have caused me to progress to liver failure and subsequent death within a few short years. I found it hard to process all this information in one go, and I think that is why he directed this part of the consultation to John. I had no doubt I would do everything in my power to survive this journey, and if that meant sticking toxic chemicals into my body, I knew I would do it.

Tears welled up in my eyes and streaked my cheeks, and I momentarily lost my train of thought. My eyes refocused, and I was able to continue the conversation, even when my treacherous tears spilled over my eyelids and blurred my vision. I used to think crying was a sign of weakness, then again, I seemed to be doing more and more of it lately. Irrational tears flooded my eyes regularly, especially on my solitary morning runs. Did that make me weak? I didn't think so.

I couldn't even glance at John. I was afraid that if I did, I would lose what little composure I had. I couldn't afford to lose it now, not in this crucial moment. John acknowledged and recognized my pain. He placed his hand on my knee and squeezed it gently.
I still needed answers. The fundamental question for me was about my son. Had I infected him? Tears cascaded down my face and throat, soaking my white shirt as I tried to speak, each word caught in the intense heat of my conviction. Fire crept slowly up my neck as the burning question rose to my lips and exploded between us

He offhandedly handed me a tissue from the box on his desk, and continued to explain that the risks were low. There was still a small risk, (2-5% chance), that he may have contracted it from me during the birthing process. I asked whether he should be tested. His response was to ask me if I considered it to be worth the stress right now. Nothing could be done for him as he was not old enough to access the treatments. A thick blanket of disgrace covered me from head to toe as I processed this fact. How could I have done this to my innocent child?!

Our consultation was over. I was sent directly to the hospital to commence treatment. I barely distinguished the words as they buzzed in my ears. I comprehended every single note, but I failed to hear the music that was supposed to accompany them. I reflected on my life. Would there be a future for me now? If so, what would it look like? I once again questioned why this was happening to me, to us? A voice silently struggled within me. It desperately wanted to cry out, but I completely suppressed it. I couldn't bring forth the words I wanted to say. I was too ashamed and too embarrassed about the predicament I had placed us in.

My mind flaunted scenarios of John's utter disgust in me. I saw John as he enjoyed a happier, more fruitful and less risky life. A better life could be his, without me. I was the only obstacle. At that moment, I wished I was a mind reader, just to glean what was going on in his mind. What was he thinking about? How did he feel about me? Was he angry? Did he hate me? Did he feel trapped in this relationship? I would never know what thoughts passed through his mind, because I never asked any of these questions. The pain of knowing far outweighed the possibility of any positive responses he may have provided me.

"Worry never robs tomorrow of its sorrow; it only saps today of its strength."

- A. J. Crown

Chapter 68

My reflection

I can't tell you exactly when I first contracted HCV. During my life, I have received unscreened blood products, such as the Rhesus injections after the birth of my children in the early '80s and '90s, I have had surgical procedures, been part of mass school vaccination programs and lived and received medical treatment in Papua New Guinea. However, I do believe it was probably 20 odd years ago, when I was self-indulgent and experimental in my youthful years, although I cannot remember ever sharing any injecting equipment. I was careful even back then, but I cannot remember if I shared any of the other paraphernalia, like the swabs, tourniquet, spoon or the water. So I cannot be entirely sure how I contracted this disease, not that it really matters either way, at the end of the day I was still infected and I wasn't looking to blame anyone.

They say youth is wasted on the young. Well, my younger years were spent feeling infallible and indestructible. I held a watertight conviction that my life would perpetually roll on regardless of my antics. I never contemplated or even discussed the idea of contracting a disease from acts of sharing injecting equipment. How would I have known back then that my historical actions would bring harm to me today, twenty years later?

Those days long gone, a portion of history swept away by time, forever discarded, securely locked away where no one could access or change them. They were painful and tumultuous times for me to dwell upon. Days I would rather forget than reflect upon. But, here I was being punished for something I did back when I was young and impetuous. How could I not think about that time and what had transpired, when here I was experiencing the consequences? Look at the outcome and the carnage my bygone actions caused! The personal suffering I now forced upon not only myself but my family and friends as well. If I could take it back, I would, but this is not an option for anyone.

Chapter 69

Adversity is the best teacher
"My great concern is not whether you have failed, but whether you are content with your failure."
- Abraham Lincoln

The silent thirty minute drive to the hospital made it possible for me to reflect and compartmentalise the words that careened through my tightly-wound head. The amount of circulating virus in my body was extensive. The fact that I had cirrhosis staggered me. The whole scenario was surreal. It confounded me. I didn't display any symptoms or show any signs of being ill at all.

Cirrhosis generally manifests with overall fatigue, body aches, mental sluggishness, headaches and nausea, but I exhibited none of these symptoms. I did feel tightness over my right side, and sometimes pain, but not enough to slow me down. If you consider the damage to my liver, then I should have experienced some major bodily manifestation, but I didn't.

This latest crisis was unbelievable, incomprehensible, to me. I felt like I was in a scene from a horror film. The most terrifying event would soon be revealed. A deadly virus persistently prowled and circulated throughout my mortal body, a hidden killer, unidentified by its host for the last twenty years. It concealed itself and lurked inside me, its aim to haunt and slowly destroy its prey, me.

The ongoing tragedy of living unaware of a hidden killer was the heartbreak of unknowingly putting those I dearly loved and others at risk. The prospect of this, should it occur, would be my grand finale, my final scene. I could not live with that on my conscience. I knew that household transmission was extremely low unless our bloods mixed from sharing toiletries et cetera. Still, my husband and I had been in some high risk situations, and, thankfully, he wasn't infected. I thanked God for this saving Grace.

Life is so fragile, a mirror so easily broken. As I pondered my situation, I became conscious of the fact I had taken my life for granted, thinking I would live forever. How naïve was I?! I had always believed, the secret to reaping the greatest fruit was to live on the edge. This philosophy fit perfectly with my nature. However, I now knew that my perspectives were all wrong, and that by living my life dangerously, I was now living the consequences of my actions.

This challenging stumble I had taken had most likely prevented a potentially major fall. I may have never found out about my condition, and contracted liver cancer or liver failure. I needed to look at my situation from another angle. There was always good mixed with the bad, and I needed to focus on the positive aspects. This bitter trial I faced was really a blessing in disguise. It could have saved my life.

One of my biggest regrets was that I had not lived a healthier lifestyle. I was unaware of the potential dangers of drinking even the smallest amount of alcohol. The potentially fatal affects it can have on a struggling liver are immense. Aussies are big drinkers, we socialise regularly, and I was no different. I had most likely contributed to my cirrhosis by my heavy bouts of drinking in my twenties, and then the years of the odd glass of wine with dinner or a few cocktails at a nightclub had most likely fast tracked my liver disease.

I did eat well, more vegetarian than 'carnivore', what I would call a diet full of meat. I ate a diet full of fresh juices, fruit and vegetables, with the occasional meat dish. Maybe this is what kept me symptom free all these years, I don't know.

"To forgive is to set a prisoner free and discover that the prisoner was you."

Lewis B. Smedes

Chapter 70

Labelled for all to see
'Nothing is so strong as gentleness, and nothing is so gentle as true strength".
St. Francis De Sales

The hospital materialized before us, bricks and mortar with coloured large lettered signs which directed us towards the parking area. We parked the car and sat, silently contemplating our surroundings. Internally, I questioned what treatment would hold for me? A cure? How would it affect me? Could I really go through with it? How sick would I become? Would I be able to work? I couldn't dwell on these questions, as they made me nervous.

I gathered all the necessary paperwork, ready to commence my battle. A war was about to begin against my unwanted passenger. John grabbed my hand and we started on our new quest. He had become the scaffolding in my life, the substance that held me together, especially in these dark hours. I don't think I could have travelled this road without him.

Together, we walked down a long, active, yet sterile, corridor. Lively people in nurse's uniforms hustled apprehensive patients into busy waiting rooms. We were ushered into a large, overcrowded room. I noticed a large reception area with a counter covered in numerous colourful advertisements where administration officers bundled and sorted through piles of patient files and sat answering phones and directing new clients. The reception desk unashamedly advertised this was a HCV clinic, and this was my destination.

I felt naked amongst the large crowd. Shame shrouded me. It blanketed me with menopausal-like hot flushes which turned my face pink. Feelings of awkwardness and humiliation manifested. I focused on the ugly tiled floor as a confident, yet emotionally colour blind, nurse gathered my paperwork and asked the final questions.

She pointed to another waiting area and we were once again instructed to sit and wait. I noticed people from all walks of life as they lingered and passed time, waiting and assessing each other. My heart rapidly thumped in my chest as I felt critiqued by my fellow comrades, the depth of my shame was, I thought, obvious to everyone present.

A deep, throaty voice echoed my name around the room. I looked up. A stern, detached nurse sought me. She offhandedly handed me a jar and told me she required a urine sample for drug testing. My whole body flinched. A urine sample? I couldn't believe it. I wanted to disappear, shrivel up into a ball so the searing stares of the onlookers wouldn't remain focussed on me.

I looked at her horrified. What was she insinuating? I wanted to scream at her, to tell her I had not touched any drugs in over twenty years! I hardly ever took a Panadol, let alone drugs. I was mute. Words streamed from my brain to my lips, but I would not allow them to be released. They would be imprisoned forever. The truth had been stated and my name had been called. I was labelled a drug addict in front of the whole room.

My legs progressively moved in the direction of the bathroom. My tense body produced an automated sample and I secretly handed her the plastic tightly-capped jar. She stood in the waiting room beside a small, white-covered table with my sample in her hand. Right there out in the open, she unscrewed the plastic container and proceeded to test its contents! I felt exposed and humiliated when she told me my sample was clear. She then directed us down the long hall to an empty room, where we were told to take a seat. She then informed us that someone would be along shortly. I was too shocked to care about her manner or anything else anymore.

The words of a song my brothers band created rang in my ears, "I am your refuge, put your hand in mine, and I will show you the way. I can heal your troubled heart and your life of disarray, all I'm asking is for you to put your hand in mine. When your strength is gone and the storms rage, listen closely and you will hear my voice. I am asking, but it's still your choice to put your hand in mine, and I will show you the way. I can make a brighter day." I had to focus on the words, and I continue to place my situation in God's hands. I had absolutely nothing to lose. My life was out of my control now anyway.

We waited in an uninviting, clinical-looking room. It had a large television strategically placed in front of two of the three plastic chairs, and an oversized table sat in the corner. This formal, inexpressive room provided freedom from the noise, freedom from the inquisitors prying eyes, and freedom from their eavesdropping. It also offered me a space to assemble my thoughts and prepare myself for treatment.

My life was in checkmate, my king caught by the dark knight. I was unable to move. My life was completely overpowered. I was like a piece on the chess board, a pawn to be manoeuvred at will by others. As I sat waiting, I realised I was defeated in every way.
John sat quietly beside me, waiting. Looking at him made me feel more humiliated, more demeaned, yet somehow, humbled. He was here ready to take the journey with me.

Ultimately, on the other side of this voyage, lay a freedom from HCV. I needed to focus on how I would use that freedom. I knew what I had to do to get there, the long road of treatment, forty-eight weeks' worth. I knew it would be a solitary, hard journey; one only I could endure. John would support me, but I wondered if I possessed the strength to see it through? Doubts, like traitors, threatened my resolve in this final hour.

I was about to relinquish the reigns of my health and surrender my life into the hands of another, all of which left a bitter taste in my mouth. I had to completely rely on my doctor, and have ultimate faith in his expertise, judgment and skills if I was to beat HCV. My faith in the doctor, and my faith in God, I hoped would be enough to get me through the next nine months.

Time passed and still no words transpired between John and I. Silence thickened the atmosphere. Out of the blue, a woman entered the room, she offhandedly introduced herself, switched on the video player, told us someone else would attend to us for the treatment segment, and walked out again.

So many faces, no continuity. No wonder people don't understand the process, or the disease. John tilted his head towards mine. Our foreheads softly united. Our cheerless eyes met in a heartbreaking moment of connection. He curved his eyebrows into a comical expression, and in a quirky tone said, "great bedside manner." His attempt at humour, in these circumstances, made me laugh and it broke the tension between us.

I knew I was held in the arms of someone who knew my every need, and there wasn't anywhere else I wanted to be. The video continued to play. Its educational contents were a monotonous, boring script. The ceaseless humming of the overhead, bright fluorescent lights distracted both of us. The video stopped and we sat and stared at the blank screen. I slowly processed the information I had been given. A calm stillness fell over the room. I knew I could not do it. It was physically and mentally impossible for me to plunge a syringe into the fleshy part of my stomach. I was needle-phobic. What was I going to do? Panic rose up within me. I tried to speak, to tell John I couldn't go through with it, but before I could, John discerned my internal turmoil. He grabbed my hand and unflinchingly stated he would do it for me.

He had been privy to my fears, and understood the private pain I now felt. Together, we had weathered many storms. We were seasoned partners who could anticipate each other's moves. We took refuge in each other's arms when the seas were rough, and he knew I was in the midst of a personal typhoon, a rough patch, and he would step up to the bridge and take over, because he understood I was incapable.

The door flung open. A smiling, dark-haired woman strode confidently in, her arms full of bags and paperwork. She plonked her items on the table in the corner, then sat in the vacant chair and faced us. I thought, "she's got the wrong room!"

She introduced herself as the treating doctor, and her name went in my ear and straight out the other one. "Okay, here we go," I thought. Her open manner and warm friendly smile put me at ease immediately. She moved quickly through the process of treatment, and then it was time to prepare the syringe and start. Just these words made my heart race and the muscles in my legs go rigid and tense. Acid in my stomach fought to stay in its place as nausea made my head swoon. I had an overwhelming sensation to run, as well as vomit. I still didn't think I could do it. My mind and body fought against each other, words against actions as they collided in a battle zone.

As a yoga teacher, I had practised meditation skills. I had learnt how to take my mind away from what the physical body experienced. I summoned images I knew would calm me. My therapeutic thoughts turned to the beach. I brought forth the sound of the waves as they gently crashed onto the shore. I felt the warmth of the sun as it caressed my skin and the gritty sand twisted and clustered between my toes. I visualised the colour and the coolness of the water as it splashed up my bare legs, and I could smell the salt as it clung in the air. I held tightly to this vision and a peaceful aura washed over me.

However, I was brought back to reality of the situation when I noticed the contents of the blue Pegasys bag on the table before me. In front of me lay an oversized hard plastic placemat with a yellow sharps container and alcohol swabs, and the dreaded pre-filled syringe lay before me. The thing was basically ready to go, preloaded. My eyes lingered on it. I momentarily visualised the tip as it sharply pierced the layers of fat on my stomach. I started to sweat. I felt waves of panic swell like the waves, and I felt the pull of the rip as it threatened to drag me under.

Once again, I silently cried out to God, "why was this happening to me? Was this my punishment? Was there any way out? Do I really have to go through all this?" I started to think about the promises in the Bible about healing. "Why wouldn't He heal me?" I asked, I pleaded, I didn't want to have to go through this suffering if I didn't have to. I was caught up in the surging questions. I had to stop and get some control, so I shut my ears tight, unwilling to hear what the doctor said. I wanted all this over with and me to be far away from here and this situation...

My thoughts were fractured by words of instruction. I was told to lie on the bed, face up. Under the watchful eye of the doctor, my husband prepared the scene. He lay out all the instruments, swabbed my stomach, looked for the bevelled tip, placed it on my stomach then plunged it in. Finally it was over, my first injection completed, and the long journey of treatment had begun.

"Laughter is good medicine for the soul. Our world is desperately in need of more medicine."

- Jim Stovall

Chapter 71

Passing through the flames unaffected

> *"To wish to be well is part of becoming well."*
> *- Seneca*

The doctor explained I would most likely feel quite ill when I awoke in the morning. I may experience headaches and nausea, maybe a few body aches and a slight temperature, a bit like having a touch of the flu. We were instructed to administer the interferon injections every Friday for the next forty-eight weeks, and the other tablets, the ribavirn, I was to take five of daily, two in the morning and three at night. These reportedly caused anaemia, which is lowered levels of haemoglobin, red cells, and could result in shortness of breath and a cough, but my doctor would monitor my progress. Then we were sent home, and once again I realised my perception was a lot worse than the actual event.

I went to bed that night a little apprehensive, expecting the worst to happen. Before the healing power of sleep could take me, I lay on the bed with my eyes open as I replayed the day's events. I weighed up what may occur in the morning, when I got up. I wondered what would happen. How sick would I get? What would I say to people? I wouldn't be able to hide the fact that I may be sick for a long time. I had to work out some sort of strategy. Never the less, the journey had begun and all would be revealed with the dawning of the new day.

I had passed through the flames and rose through the ashes, with not a single symptom. I rolled over and poked my partner in the ribs and jokingly blamed him for not injecting me properly. I wasn't about to waste a day, so I rallied my running partners and off we went. It was like nothing had happened, nothing had changed. I felt great.

Once again, I was blessed. My testimony is not like others, as I did not suffer from any of the signs and symptoms that most people get when they are on treatment. I have spoken to people that have been so sick they have not been able to get out of bed, let alone go to work or go through the daily functions of life.

I have to say, treatment didn't really disrupt my daily life at all. Well, not in the beginning, anyway. I did a few things that may have positively helped me. One of which was to seek Naturopathic advice and treatment shortly after my diagnosis. The naturopath I chose was someone I knew and had worked for previously. He was well-educated and had been practicing a long time. I had great faith in his abilities and he was sympathetic to my plight.

He started me on a regime of supplements including ginger tea, liver herbs, high doses of vitamin C, hormone supports and vitamin B supplements. I continued on this regime all the way through my treatment. I believe it was his help as well as my strong constitution and faith that minimised my side effects.

The first four weeks passed with little disruption to my life, except for the despised weekly injections that my husband administered. I was infected with two strains of Genotype one (1a1b). Unfortunately Genotype I is the hardest to cure and requires the longest treatment regime of forty-eight weeks. I had prepared myself mentally for that, but I was totally unprepared for the barrage of blood tests that accompanied treatment, such as the week two, four, eight, twelve, sixteen, twenty I think... You get the picture. At the end of it, you feel like a pin cushion.

> *"In the end, life lived to its fullest is its own Ultimate Gift."*
>
> *- Jim Stovall*

Chapter 72

Facades needed and worn
"Never, never, never give up."
Winston Churchill

I reached week twelve quite uneventfully, still able to work, run and going through the motions of living a normal life, all without any significant side effects. At week twelve, I was required to have another PCR test, to assess whether or not the treatment was successful.

I tried not to focus on the fact that I needed a miracle to clear this virus. I was not the best candidate. I was overweight, over forty, living with a high viral load, and to top it all off, I had cirrhosis. But I had created a plan, and I intended to follow it through till the end, and I would do everything in my power to beat it.

I needed my blood test to show a large drop, or even better, an undetectable viral load. If this was not the case, I would be removed from the treatment program. I would have no other options, but to live my life to the best of my abilities, being regularly monitored for cancer markers and subtle changes in my liver profile. There was no naturopathic or alternative cure available to me at that time.

There was a two week wait for my test results, and it was a difficult time. Each day was a laborious task where internal turmoil grew within me. I was hopelessly consumed with my need to be set free from the tight girdle that constricted my life. I desperately wanted my life back. I hated the way I felt about myself. HCV made me feel disgusting and black inside, and I wanted those feeling to go.

To the world, I used the right words. I wore an optimistic mask for all to see, but I couldn't deceive myself, my own personal, pessimistic pantomime continued. My acting ability pathetic, from my view, but to everyone else realistic, as it convinced many that I was coping well. I spoke meaningless words, none of which I believed would come to fruition. I knew the truth. The words I spoke held no real meaning for me, because I knew I didn't deserve to be freed from my internal hell. This was my punishment for all the wrong I had done throughout my life.

The results returned and displayed what I already believed. I was still infected, but my viral load had dropped dramatically. This meant the treatment was working, just not as quickly as the doctor had hoped. I was instructed to continue on treatment for another twelve weeks and the tests would be repeated at week twenty-four. I was sceptical but hopeful at the same time. It was working. I could see that. Deep inside me, at night before sleep would take me, I screamed to the heavens and dreamed of hope, with no real belief or faith that it would actually occur.

I allowed a small ray of sunshine to trickle down to where I waited in my pit. Would it work? Was I worthy enough? Did I dare to dream that it would? Would I be healed? Would I be given a second chance? If I was, I would try to make a difference, and I would use this gift wisely.

When something beyond reason occurs, it has the potential to turn sceptics into believers. I wasn't a sceptic, but my faith was weak. I believed that a higher power, my God, wanted me to continue on this road trip. So I continued and wondered what the outcome would be.

"Keep your fears to yourself, but share your courage with others".

- Robert Louis Stevenson

Chapter 73

Continual commitment
"Some people, no matter how old they get, never lose their beauty. They merely move it from their faces into their heart."
- Martin Buxbaum

A monotonous exchange of tablets, followed by the Friday injections, occurred. Circles of red, raised ridges camouflaged the lightly coloured skin on my belly, caused by the Interferon. My live-in supporter, John, found it hard to access a new injection site, without having to go over the evidence of its predecessor.

The treatment regime and John's dedication taught me about real love. They taught me about trust and acceptance and to accept who I was. I knew with clarity that John loved me and would stand beside me throughout this ordeal. His acts constantly demonstrated his enduring patience, his genuine concern, and his continual commitment to seeking a healthy, positive outcome for us both. He believed we would make it, and he had hope. A hope that lived and burned deep in my soul also, and longed to be allowed to surface, but I dared not fully unleash it, as I knew that disappointment would crush me.

During the next twelve weeks, I learnt to really pray. I learnt to speak to my higher power like a friend. I cried with Him, I laughed with Him, but mostly I talked with him about my fears and frustrations. I found payer to be a haven from my inner turmoil. I used it when I was angry, when I was frustrated, when I was scared, but mostly when fear threatened to take me. It opened my mind and my heart, and led me to others, who wanted to support me. However, at the back of my mind, I still doubted that God would totally accept me. I was after all, a joke. I certainly didn't think I deserved His attention. But, I sought it anyway, simply because I had no other option.

In the Garden of Eden, man was given one commandment, don't eat the fruit, but it was consumed anyway, and it resulted in a fall from grace. I had broken every single one of the Ten Commandments

Moses was given, so how could I possibly be worthy of any consideration. I wouldn't be surprised if I was banished to the ends of the earth.

The problem was, I felt I had nowhere else to go. I felt trapped. I was like a wounded lioness. I had been struck a blow that left me injured, alone and starving on the savannah. What were my options? I was humbled and I needed help if I was to survive the rugged terrain that surrounded me, and my wounds needed time to heal.

> *"Ultimately you are doing what you do for one of two reasons: to serve oneself or to serve God."*
>
> *- Unknown*

Chapter 74

A wounded lioness
"Our lives begin to end the day we become silent about things that matter."
- Rev. Martin Luther King, Jr

Towards the end of week twenty-four, I had begun to feel lethargic. My appetite had decreased, and I had developed a cough, as well as a painful red rash on the back of my knees. I continued to exercise every second day, but found that if I ran my usual five kilometres, I had to lay down breathless for a few hours afterwards, to recover. I changed my diet, and started to substitute food for a lot of fruit and vegetable juices and soy-based protein smoothies. I struggled to provide my body with optimum nutrients, whilst I slowly poured a stream of chemicals into it, my daily dose of kryptonite. Weight started to fall from my body. Those stubborn kilos I thought I would never lose were being shed quite rapidly.

Week twenty-four crept thoughtlessly into my existence. It brought a new sense of anxiety and apprehension. The mandatory tests had been requested, and were now completed. This was it. I would have my answer. Would I be cured, or would I be left to fend for myself on the desolate savannah?

We nervously sat again, at the specialist's office. This was a critical space in time, filled with fervent hope. Would the results show I have no virus left, or would it show the opposite? I contemplated the questions I wanted to ask. I systematically created a mental list. Previously answered questions bounced around in my head. I felt like a ticking time bomb. Raw emotions ascended to the surface and my desperation was evident for the whole world to see.

Living with this virus felt like the sun setting over the feeding ground on the plains. The darkness allowed the lowly scavengers time to slither around my body and destroy me cell by cell. Night is great for the hunters, but not for the hunted, and I felt like I was the hunted. I knew that if I didn't clear this virus, I would be enthusiastically stalked and prepared for the final kill.

My name was called. The specialist greeted us both at the door. He grabbed my partner's hand, shook it, leant forward and kissed me on the cheek, then ushered us into his now very familiar office. Before he had a chance to sit in his chair, I asked him if I was able to continue on treatment.

He turned to peer at me over the rims of his spectacles. Over the past six months, I had grown to really like and trust this man, he was honest, open and upfront. We had many debates and discussions about testing procedures, disease progression and upcoming new treatments. The latest theories were always a hot topic between us. He didn't always agree with where my research took me, especially when I discussed O-zone therapy in the USA. We debated this subject in-depth. He listened intently to my latest findings, then composedly and solemnly informed me that people were dying from blood poisoning, to which I had no response.

He also didn't agree with my faith in natural therapies, often commenting to my partner about it being a waste of money. I believed there was a place for all types of medicine, and complementary medicine had in my mind been proven time and time again, even when conventional medicine had failed.

It was my life and I had to choose what I thought was best for me. It was up to me to navigate through the mine field of predators out there in the world. This lioness was not about to change her mind on her choice to utilise the skills of the natural therapist in combination with the current course of chemotherapy.

> *"We shall draw from the heart of suffering itself the means of inspiration and survival."*
>
> ***Sir Winston Churchill***

Chapter 75

Words can penetrate armour
"Failure is not an event, but rather a judgment about an event. Failure is not something that happens to us or a label we attach to things. It is a way we think about outcomes."
- John Ortberg

He sat down and faced me, crossed his arms over his chest and informed me that I had not been able to clear the virus. A silence reigned over us whilst I digested the information. I knew what this meant. I was going off treatment. I had no other options. He could do nothing further for me except monitor my liver progression and hopefully catch a potential cancer before it was inoperable.

I felt frozen, anesthetized. A pitch black night descended upon me. Its bitter coldness, seeped deep into my bones. I was back at square one, the wind gone, completely removed from my sails. I was speechless. That hidden, compressed hope was now squashed, replace by devastation.

I thought I had tamed the beast within me, discarded it, but it slowly made its presence known to me as it invaded me, like an uninvited cancer. It spread subtly but thoroughly throughout my body, saturating my being in hopelessness. I had valiantly fought, but lost the battle. I would leave here, once again defeated, the glory to be offered to someone else. A revelation I didn't want to hear.

My mind shut down. I was unable to process any more of the soundless words that fell from his lips. My resolve had been weakened. My eyes faded, and the floor became my primary focus. I thought I was prepared for those words, but I wasn't. I thought I had equipped myself for this day, but in reality, I hadn't. Anguish hits some harder than others, and I was literally shattered.

As I sat in his office, I realised that I secretly anticipated I would beat it. I had come to truly believe in the lie I told others. I believed I had a fighting chance. All my acting and bravado was an actual audition for the real deal, a part I didn't receive, but secretly believed

I would. I recounted every day. I knew I had adhered to the treatment regime stringently, not missing one day. I ruminated over questions I dared not ask. What could have gone wrong? What did I do wrong? What would happen now? The answers scared me.

I couldn't move or speak. I sat motionless, like a petrified statue. I felt a pressure on my hand, as it was totally engulfed. I felt like I was becoming mentally unstable. A big burden weighed heavy on me, and it defeated me. A panic stricken voice spoke beside me, rousing me from my oppression, "what happens now?" I knew monitoring was my only option. I would be required to have an ultrasound every six months and more blood tests to assess cancer markers – alpha feta protein tests. This was hardly the reassurance John desired. He wanted more conviction, more certainty, but it was not offered, as it wasn't the truth.

I felt like a loose cannon. My mind triggered explosive muscle responses, and negative thought processes blasted over my synapses. I needed to refocus and get some perspective. I needed to stop and draw a deep breath. Relax my body. Control my emotions. I needed to pull myself together. I drew a big, deep breath, and pure cool air filled my body. It transported a calming effect to every cell, It soothed me and brought clarity back to my mind. My concentration centred back on the doctor. I could see his sympathy and sincerity as it was demonstrated in his words and written on his face. He explained that the treatment had decreased the viral load, and provided my liver with time to heal, so all was not in vain.

Feelings of failure became the centre of my attention. They overrode any motivation to seek or consider alternative treatments. I couldn't see any other options right now. The horizon that once held such promise and beauty was now empty and distant.

I briefly inquired about the new treatments - the protease inhibitors; however, I already knew they were not an option. They were still years away from being placed on the market. Whilst my husband and the specialist debated success rates, my mind drifted internally. My eyes glazed over and I mentally transported myself to my safe place, the peaceful, undisturbed, quiet beach.

I was roused from my serenity, by my husband inquiring if I was alright. My voice refused to surface, my eyes glued to the floor. I slowly nodded in agreement, not able to meet his eyes, for fear they would betray me. The conversation rang around me like loud, tolling church bells, a constant rambling sound, in which nothing was discernible.

Our time was up. Unanswered questions, like a bright red lipstick, lingered on my lips. As I stood ready to leave, I asked if I was going to make another five years. He explained that studies demonstrated that people who go on HCV treatment live longer and also have lower incidences of liver cancer, so, most likely yes, but there were no guarantees in life.

"You may not realize it when it happens, but a kick in the teeth may be the best thing in the world for you".

Walt Disney

Chapter 76

Entombed

> *"Remember, you may choose your sin, but you cannot choose the consequences."*
> **-Jenny Sanford**

The drive home was speechless. The window offered solace as the world swiftly sped past me. I was inarticulate, words adrift in the turbulent sea of my thoughts. My inability to focus tilted my world off course, chaos began to establish itself, and despondency took up residence. I refused to meet John's periodic gaze, which regularly probed me for answers I couldn't provide. During the silent drive, I saw harrowing motion pictures depicting my impending death. Words directed me to leave the family, to run away, and die somewhere on my own.

I didn't want to coexist with a virus for the rest of my life. I didn't think I could. I found myself again, asking God WHY? This punishment was rather extreme, I thought. A lifetime of torment the price for a small window of time misspent. How could I now live with my family? How could I make love to my husband? I couldn't see how I could live a normal life anymore. I felt unclean, dirty, rotting away from the inside out. I asked myself if it was all worth it?

No, I didn't think so.

I planned my diversion, my getaway. I made up my mind not to put my family in any more risk. I would leave and allow them the opportunity to live a normal, happy life; hopefully a gratifying life, without the constant threat of infection from what lurked inside me. I wanted them to move on, without me. As painful as I knew it would be, I also rationalised that this option was the best for everyone...

I started to sabotage my relationship with John, and it didn't take long to spiral downwards. I pulled away from him, locking him out, unable and unwilling to share any of my feelings. I couldn't share what I didn't understand. I found myself living in the land of the lost. I had become a severely injured lioness, flanked by millions of tiny predators, waiting whilst my will to live ebbed away each day. I wanted the solid ground beneath me to open up and swallow me, and it did.

I was buried whilst still living. A coffin of conviction imprisoned me. It held me deep in the ground. I felt completely submerged; the protective garments I once wore were now discarded on the surface. I lay entombed within myself, and allowed the darkness to totally seize the worthy and enjoyable portions of my life and place dark shadows over them.

A small light flickered far above me. My local GP called to see how I was. He left a message for me, and I went to see him. I sat and cried in his office whilst I offloaded my plight. He listened intently then gently patted me on the hand. He told me he would order more tests, and then we could make some real decisions. The unbearable weight of the ground above me shifted slightly. I had not thought of that. The test would take a few days, and I found myself waiting again for results.

"Laughter is the sun that drives winter from the human face."

- Victor Hugo

Chapter 77

Darkness prevails

"What you leave behind is not what is engraved in stone monuments, but what is woven into the lives of others."
- Pericles

It was the middle of winter, cold and dark. The 4am alarm droned from the wooden bedside table. John slowly, noisily, rolled out of bed to go to work. His movement roused me from my disturbed sleep. As soon as I woke up, my mind became fully alert, ready to go.

My internal cinema automatically switched to fast forward, and displayed visions of death, funerals, family, suffering, isolation and regret. Self-loathing and condemnation lived alongside me. They had become squatters in my life, now my constant roommates.

Overwhelming desires to pack up, run and give in, detonated around me like strategically planted bombs. I couldn't work out what had happened to me. I knew I couldn't go on like this. These thoughts would ruin me if they continued

I slipped out of bed, believing that a change of scenery would stop my self-imposed harassment. I snuggled deep into the soft lounge chair, and waited for the sun to lighten my world. Hours passed as I pondered and meditated on my circumstances.

Daylight trickled into the room, and I moved into the dining room. I found myself alone in the quietness of a familiar, yet unchanging, motionless house as my son made his own way to school. The sun sparkled playfully through the open blinds. Its shadows danced and flaunted themselves on the large wooden table, where I sat. The warmth of the day touched me, heating my face. It conveyed a calming presence. The ambience was peaceful and serene.

Nevertheless, my thoughts were dark and sinister. I found my vision was much sharper and clearer in the shadowy world, where it now regularly dwelt.

My dark thoughts turned ominously to the end. I already knew it was better for everyone if I was taken out of the equation. If I ran away to Cairns, that wouldn't give anyone closure, but my death would. I believed they would all be able to move on in life if that occurred. An unedited funeral played out before me. One I had visually created and planned in great detail. I knew I could easily implement it. I would no longer make promises to anyone, because I knew I wouldn't keep any of them. I had made my decision. I had nothing to lose as my life was already over.

On the table lay a large notepad and a black pen. They waited for my instructions. My steady hand automatically commenced writing. Unwavering clear words filled the paper with an uncontrolled compulsion. My own funeral service was created in full detail with clear instructions. The curtain was now drawn on my life. My demons had won. I had relinquished my life, and here it lay in black and white. I was surprised how little time this task took, how easy it was. The final feature film I had produced consumed me for hours. It was a perfect example of how effortlessly I could consider ending it all. No food or drink passed my lips as the final preparations were made.

The wrench of the three o'clock school pick up broke my self-absorbed trance. It forced me to resurface from my six hour obsession. Realisation struck me; I couldn't believe I had spent all day visualising and playing out my own death. How macabre! It was then I knew something was very wrong with me. Generally in my darkest moments, my kids were my guiding light, but their bulbs had blown, and the lighthouse that once guided me was empty, devoid of any radiance. Darkness now prevailed where their light had once been.

I always thought that if you played a role long enough, the role would somehow become real. However my performance as a laisser-faire, happy go lucky human being, was not the role I now chose.

> *"Nothing could be worse than the fear that one had given up too soon, and left one unexpended effort that might have saved the world."*
> *Jane Addams*

Chapter 78

My vision clears
"Relying on God has to start all over every day, as if nothing has yet been done."
-C.S.Lewis

My son, now at home, settled comfortably into his natural routine. I decided to go for a long walk to finalise the details of my plan. I wanted it all to end. For me, the deal was done, written on a notepad which sat on the table. Everything was clear and settled in my heart and I was ready and willing to hand my life over.

As I walked, I wondered what could bring me to this place. Was this depression? How could I be fine last week, and feel so different today? I was actually contemplating the end of my life? What was wrong with me? I held a strong belief that suicide was wrong. The thought of spending eternity in a place I didn't want to be frightened me. But, other more sinister feelings plagued me and overruled any belief systems I had.

Could the treatment I had just finished do this to me? I recalled one of the side effects was depression. But, what I was feeling was so intense, so real, so powerful and so consuming. Was that depression? Would I succumb to it? Would I be overcome by the internal demons that overshadowed my convictions and my principles? Was I strong enough to resist the temptation, to take the easy option, which was continually flaunted in my face?

Walking, like running, always released my mind from its prison cell, and today my stave of execution was granted. The further I walked, the more I became liberated from the overpowering, crushing reflections that had held me captive all day. My vision cleared. A new icon rallied under the spotlight, anger.

I started to yell and scream at God. Words I will not repeat here. I was angry, furious with Him, for allowing this to happen. Visions of starving, emaciated children who suffered throughout the world immediately flooded my awareness. Fleetingly, I felt guilty for my thoughts, but I was so self-consumed, I easily ignored these mental pictures. I needed help, and I needed someone to help me, otherwise it was over for me. Rivulets of tears streaked my windblown face, as I loudly and furiously yelled into the void. I can't do this anymore! Just take me! Take me now!

Through my ranting and my anger, I felt tranquillity fall. A quite peaceful calm covered me. I stood in the eye of a cyclone, whilst debris floated around me. Words and phrases both spoken and unspoken encircled me, trapped in the raging winds. A name dropped with the torrent of rain. An omen. She was a woman I had not had contact with for many years. I wondered if she was still around.

I momentarily ceased walking, stunned. Did that really just happen, or did I imagine it? Did I hear it correctly? I think someone actually spoke to me. Was that God, instructing me? Yes, I think it could have been. I could not feel any lower than I felt right now. I was in the gutter, ruined and consumed with my own self-pity. I knew this was my last chance. I realised my hope had been tragically misplaced.

My father had always said that God claims his children in the final hour. This was my final hour. Every step homeward brought me a little more strength, a little more courage. A new attitude formed. It rose slowly from the ashes of the decaying world I had placed myself in.

My house came into view, and as I looked at it, it beckoned me. It reached out for me and invited me to stay. As I looked at it, I felt encouraged, as my history was mingled with the paint on its walls. I stood for a few moments and stared at its familiarity. I felt I needed to rise up and be the woman I was supposed to be. I needed to be strong, for today was not the day for giving in or running away. I realised I wasn't prepared to throw my life away, not today. But, if I was to keep living, I would need to start to really fight for my place here on this earth. I had allowed my enemies to get a foothold in my life. A battle of self-control and determination would need to be waged, and hopefully, it would build strength of character. I vowed,

I would never place myself in this situation ever again.

I simply wasn't strong enough to fight this battle, except........ I had been given a name, a saviour, a friend, a helper, to overcome the dark moments. Finally, I felt someone was listening to me. I felt heard, and now I understood there could be another way. It didn't have to end like I had previously planned and written. I walked into my sanctuary more determined than I had been in a long time.

> *"The toys and blocks with which we play are houses, lands and gold. Their values quickly pass away, as does a tale that's told. But kindly, gracious deeds abide, their wealth will not depart; their flowers of joy are multiplied in gardens of the heart".*
>
> *- Charles Russell Wakeley*

Chapter 79

A lifeline is offered
"Continuous effort---not strength or intelligence--is the key to unlocking our potential."
-Winston Churchill

Betty was a kind, gentle, God-fearing woman. We had shared a surrogate mother-daughter relationship in another time. A strong bond of mentoring, love, trust and acceptance had once joined us but was long gone as my current path had separated us.

Oddly, as I searched the telephone directory, I found her number straight away, like it was there waiting for me all this time. Our lines of communication reopened, and her buoyant cheerful voice filled the air ways. It was like I had just seen her yesterday. She asked me what had taken me so long to call, as she had been waiting for me to make contact with her. She told me God had prepared her, as she was aware and ready for the battle ahead. She vowed to wear her armour and wield her sword and fight beside me. My heart lifted, why didn't I think to ring her sooner?

The dark, heavy veil that had shrouded my life for the last six months slowly lifted, and the battle to regain a foothold in my life began. The dark, depressing hours retreated, replaced by a new optimistic day, a path reincarnated from previous times. I experienced a new feeling of excitement and elation. I needed her now, more than ever.

I still felt scared, reluctant to go on, but her encouraging words echoed loudly in my ear. I could overcome this, but I needed to trust God. Together Betty and I focused on constructing a new road. A road I could understand and walk upon. She told me, overall success was my final destination, but really it was the journey that truly mattered. The goal was to reach the end however I needed the ability to look back and appreciate all of the bumps and potholes, as well as to walk away knowing I did the best I could.

I put the phone down. Fear no longer drove me. Hope was

resurrected, and it sat firmly in the driver's seat, taking full control. Over the following weeks, she helped me to uncover the truth. The truth that I really did have something to live for: my family and my friends. She made me realise that my life had meaning to so many others. It didn't matter what had happened, because everything has a beginning and an end. The journey is the part that teaches us life's lessons and everything in life is worth partaking of. It doesn't matter how crappy things look from the outside, something good always rises from it.

A marathon was about to begin, a long slow run that hopefully would go on for the next forty odd years. My endurance would be tested and it would be a battle all the way to the finish line. I would run the race of my life. Hopefully, my supporters would celebrate my milestones with me and congratulate me on my successes. She helped me find a new sense of purpose and made me identify that the only real legacy I had was not what others thought of me, but what God thinks. Betty gave me all this insight with just a few conversations.

I wondered why I had kept myself in the darkness for so long. Why did I think I could do this journey alone? I obviously couldn't. Look what had come to pass from my previous decisions. I was depressed, composing funeral plans! What a mess I had made of my life! I had pushed John and the rest of the family away. I sensed I needed to refocus on rebuilding my relationships, and over the next few weeks that was exactly what I did. I made them like the gears in my new vehicle. They became my priority.

Another ray of sunshine had been sent my way when I reconnected with her. The whole situation was more than I understood. It was a great mystery, but it provided immeasurable love to me in my darkest hour. Excitement and joy filled me every time I drove to meet her, all my doubts or fears replaced by acceptance and love. She would rush out to greet me before I had even locked the car. She would grab and hug me tightly like I was her long lost child.

I felt warm, loved, yearned for. She made me feel like no mountain was too big for me to climb. Only a loving mother could soothe, console and reassure injured children, and this was exactly how she made me feel. We spoke for hours as we discussed all my options and read the Bible together. We prayed and she helped me to recreate my faith into a more liveable and understandable fashion. It was awesome. I felt renewed. I became a new woman. I no longer felt defeated. I became a strong lioness that could now stalk and hunt her own prey. She helped me stand my ground. I would no longer be the hunted, but instead become the hunter.

Every time I left her presence, my emotional and physical batteries were topped up, overflowing even. I felt loved and totally accepted, not judged at all. Her words and support made me feel worthy to be on this path. Why me? I still didn't know, but I realised it no longer mattered. What mattered was what I would make of the situation. I vowed to step out in faith and win. I was ready for the next hurdle.

Unfortunately, our paths were separated when she got very ill and I couldn't see her for a while. It didn't matter, because together we had chartered a new course for me. She had provided me with the tools I needed to move forward. This was my journey, my lessons to learn, and only I could walk this path of discovery. She had equipped me and given me the strength to go on, and I would be eternally grateful to her for loving me in spite of everything.

I was thankful I had reached out to her, even if it was for a short time. She was just what I needed. She taught me to use my past experiences to correct my mistakes and to seek the future with a sense of purpose and vision, but also to cherish the moment in which I lived in, and that's exactly what I did.

"Live an honourable life. Then when you get older and think back, you'll be able to enjoy it a second time."

-Author Unknown

Chapter 80

Finding a will to fight

"What is the difference between an obstacle and an opportunity? Our attitude toward it. Every opportunity has a difficulty, and every difficulty has an opportunity."
-J. Sidlow Baxter

Shortly after devising my funeral plan and reconnecting with Betty, I took the first step on my newly chartered course, which was to get the results of the last test and review them. With Betty's help, I had made up my mind to be more proactive in my health care. What I contemplated included a trip to California for o-zone therapy, a month's stay at a health farm, or push to continue treatment.

My first step was to see the GP. I sat with my friendly Egyptian GP and we methodically reviewed the results. We discussed his findings, and I asked for his interpretation. He optimistically informed me that the treatment was definitely working. I had a dramatic drop in my viral load. My count was now under 500 copies per unit of blood, down from well over 1.5 million copies. My specialist worked under the stringent governmental guidelines, and was only able to provide ongoing treatment if my viral load was not detectable. Well, five hundred copies, to me, was nearly undetectable.

I went straight home and emailed the specialist. I asked to be put back on treatment. I followed this up with a telephone conversation the next day, and I was back on treatment within the week. I calculated I had missed no more than ten days of treatment. I was ready to diligently face another twenty-four weeks, and I was determined to complete it regimentally.

A string of days and nights passed. Small knots formed on the rope which held John and me together. They were insignificant hindrances to our path, small strains on our relationship, but not enough of a problem to cause either of us any concern. Over the last six months, we had become strongly and securely attached to the same anchor.

I embarked on the last twenty-four weeks with more enthusiasm. However, they were tougher than the previous ones. I knew I would not give in. My resolution was stronger than ever before. I needed and wanted to maintain a normal life, and this included working. So, I continued to work throughout the whole journey. However, I battled every day. I fought nausea, headaches and body aches, but the itchy red rashes drove me mad. The lethargy and erratic moods were probably the hardest symptoms to bare, but I would not give in to any of them.

*"**Defeat is not defeat unless accepted as a reality-in your own mind.**"*

Bruce Lee

Chapter 81

A gift of renewal

"Restlessness and impatience change nothing except our peace and joy. Peace does not dwell in outward things, but in the heart prepared to wait trustfully and quietly on Him who has all things safely in His hands."
- Elisabeth Elliot

My husband became a gallant defender of my health and well-being. He was a strong shield that protected me from the world. He bolstered my life with his love and support and assisted me every step of the way. Both of us hoped and prayed that I would score a victory and win this round.

Our previous love over the many years was tumultuous. It was fraught with dangerous terrain and deep wells, but this experience changed all that. It presented and validated our true potential. It revealed to us what we were capable of having. This voyage fostered a new love between us. My admiration and respect for John grew daily. He truly became the foundation of my life, his continual validation of our future enhanced my confidence and sense of worth. His selfless acts of kindness were astonishing. Incredible deeds full of love and compassion saturated my life from every angle.

My role as his wife was something that I had previously considered a temporary assignment, but now I viewed it as eternal and vitally important. It was the role of my lifetime. I now realized that my marriage was a precious gift; one I had taken for granted all these years. I vowed not to do this again. Betty had reminded me to cherish every moment, and that was what I planned to do.

The next twenty-two weeks were spent tackling and reducing the effects of the treatment. At times, I needed to decrease my ribavirn dose, due to ongoing nausea and fatigue. I found my weekends offered some relief from the tension of the three twelve-hour shifts I worked at the prison. My cheerful mask was a necessary pretence, which was hard to maintain when nausea and fatigue racked every inch of my chemical-ridden body. It was a mask I easily discarded on my journey home from work. My days off were spent in a ritualistic format, with me sprawled out on the lounge, encased in a temporary haven of blankets, as I watched movie after movie. About half way through the treatment, I found I was unable to continue working nightshifts, due to my emergent insomnia. Sleep became an ancient concept. My body forgot what a prolonged rest felt like, yet it earnestly craved the replenishment it offered.

As the journey drew to an end, I found it increasingly hard to maintain my alter ego. Treatment was taking its toll on both my body and my mind, but at the same time, I refused to allow myself to grow weak, however adverse the circumstances. I would not allow myself to be beaten in this final hour, no matter how many hits I had to take. I would not let my own mind lure me to throw in the towel, just because the fight was getting tougher, especially as my undaunted opponent stood steadfast.

As it got closer to the end, my husband and I envisaged something indescribable.

We saw a life without hepatitis C.

Chapter 82

Thor's hammer strikes a mighty blow
Life can only be understood backwards, but it must be lived forwards.
- Soren Kierkegaard

The weeks elapsed quickly to those around me. On the other hand, I was sensitive to every hour, living vicariously through the eyes of my alter ego. Every morning, I awoke and looked forward to another day, knowing that it would bring me closer to my destination: the end of treatment and hopefully an unencumbered life.

My final injection and my last day of tablets surfaced. That final day generated great delight in me. Pure satisfaction. I could say I had run the gauntlet and finished the race. I had completed it to the best of my ability. The question was, would I now be eligible for the prize? The cup of life was something I greatly desired. My coach held the results in his hand. The final outcome was about to be pronounced.

It was time to stand on the podium and receive a trophy. Would I walk away a winner, or a loser? In seconds, I would know. I tried to think positively, in tune with my inner desires, but the present reality was a sensation of physical discomfort. Would I experience a moment of ecstasy or affliction?

There was a sudden quietness in the midst of the turmoil. All eyes watched me closely as the findings were publicized. He finally spoke. The words I dreaded fell from his lips. I had not been successful. The crown I believed I had won was quickly snatched from my head. My efforts had been in vain. I had failed. I was the loser.

A state of physical discomfort and anguish poured over me, it drenched me in a painful sorrow, which surged like the tide. A freezing wind blew within me; its cold bite pierced every inch of me. A loneliness without comparison descended upon me, consuming me. I felt like I was driving on an isolated highway, towards an abandoned crossroad, in the middle of Antarctica. All my hopes, dreams and inspirations were forever lost, swept away in the merciless winds. How could I move forward now? What about my relationship?

I refused to look at John. I knew the disappointment and disbelief would show on his face. What would he think of me now? We had believed I would be healed, and here I was still infected and back at square one. What was I going to do?

Everything I believed and wanted was stolen from me. Thor's hammer slammed down upon me. It massacred every single dream with its distinct blow.

This outcome rocked my world, but I refused to allow myself to sink into the quicksand of my previous pit. I would not bow this time in submission to the persistent, internal threats to overpower and bury me again. I was stronger, more in control now, and I would not surrender my life. Not whilst there was still a fight left in me. I would find myself again, and I would re-challenge my co-host another time and in another way.

I needed time to lick my wounds and to regroup. For now, my race was run, completed.

"Make failure your teacher, not your undertaker."

Zig Ziglar

Chapter 83

Two paths, two destinies

"What afflicts us is a corruption of the heart, a turning away in the soul. Our aspirations, our affections and our desires are turned toward the wrong things. And only when we turn them toward the right things--toward enduring, noble, spiritual things--will things get better."
- John Buchanan

Over the ensuing months, I placed my feelings in a solid, sealed casket and buried them deep within myself, not allowing any of them to resurface. My vault was full of undeveloped negatives, labelled apprehension, dismay and trepidation. They were all processed, waiting to be placed in my internal album for deep storage.

I became a living symbol of a life full of guilt. I was emotionally dead like a corpse. I was broken. The race had been too intense, too long, and my endurance was spent. This time, instead of creating funeral plans I chose to escape into an illusion, a fabrication of my real life.

Over the next few years I would push myself to achieve miraculous things. I would reach the top of my chosen profession. But, I would do it like a destructive force and leave many ruins in my wake. The built-up stress and the accumulated strain of not clearing the virus caused a shift in my inner core, and my life became like an earthquake waiting to happen.

I chose to drag out the photo gallery of my previous albums and reminisce and live in my memories, rather than live in the real world. It was a way of holding onto the things I loved, without letting them go, but at the same time, not actually being a part of any of them. I told myself that withdrawing from my life in this fashion was not really running away, as I was still physically present. I believed it was not wise to be constantly present in my marriage, especially whilst there was more reason to fear than to hope in a future.

John also chose to escape by any means at his disposal. Alcohol and misrepresentation were his preferred choices. Unable to adequately withdraw into himself, he chose to disguise himself with lies and falsehoods, which provided him with a few moments of comfort. His medication of choice, alcohol, became his anaesthetic to help him endure the operation of life.

We both struggled to climb the mountain that grew between us, not as one team, but now, as single mountaineers. The terrain was steeper than either of us expected. Our previous love and devotion for each other became less abundant as time moved forward. The climate of our relationship became harsher and harsher, and it was physically too tough to endure.

The problem was, we both lost any ability to reason logically. We couldn't see anything beyond the steep ascent. We both decided to continue the climb, but chose routes that suited our own individual needs. We no longer considered the other and we opted for vastly different paths. I hiked to the summit alone. I faced and conquered large walls of frozen ice. Meanwhile, John sought refuge from the onslaught by deflecting the avalanches I sent cascading down from my rapid climb.

I left him alone on that ledge, whilst I pursued a career and a life that didn't include him. I reached the summit with no one at my side. I could no longer see any visible representation of my old self or my former life. The man who had stuck by me all those years, who had fought with me to conquer this disease, the man who had pledged his undying love and support for me, was now just a speck on the horizon. I had reached the top, but for what purpose? I realised, if there was no one to share it with, it was pointless.

Standing at the summit, I forced myself to be alone in my grief. I was able to assess my life and reflect on my choices. I reviewed what I had done with my life and what I had become. From this vantage point, I discovered unimaginable resources within and around me, but I also viewed my life in its reality. I had become a strong, resourceful, independent woman, but my life was really bleak. I had been offered a great life with John, and for a short time we had lived it, basking in the glory of our love, and once again I had sabotaged and thrown it away.

My grief and my perception overruled sound logic. Yes, I had HCV, but he loved me. He had demonstrated that time and time again, but still I doubted it. I came to understand how stupid I had been. I realised that the mess my life was in was a direct consequence of my actions, beliefs, perceptions and behaviours.

"If your success is not on your own terms, if it looks good to the world but does not feel good in your heart, it is not success at all."

Anna Quindlen

Chapter 84

A rise from the ashes
"Man will occasionally stumble over the truth, but most of the time he will pick himself up and continue on."
-Winston Churchill

Shortly after my treatment failure, I relinquished my position at the prison and accepted a state-wide project manager's position working in the blood-borne virus field. I entered this new role like a cyclone. I was hungry for more HCV knowledge and exposure to the services that supported people living with these viruses so I could eventually fight my war and feel more empowered.

I was like a disruptive wind, which brought major disturbances and stormy weather, but I really kicked some mighty goals. I threw myself into work, as it was a familiar concept, and I allowed it to consume me for quite some time. Conquering the summit didn't make me feel any better about myself, but work was the ultimate distraction from my internal convictions. For two years, I focused my heart and soul into a job that offered nothing in return, and I threw away what was truly important to me. My family and friends, as well as everything I had built, was now gone and I was alone, and I didn't really like how it felt.

This revelation dawned on me too late. I had built no life outside of my job. Communication with the only real person in my life had rapidly declined. His life encompassed his own expectations and moved forward in a different direction to mine. I now found myself on a mountainous, snow-covered, lonely ledge, as I watched in dismay as he climbed to another summit alone. I hated this disease and what it had stolen from me.

I had manipulated my work schedule so that I spent weeks away in lonely motel rooms. This offered time for me to reflect upon my life script. I often wondered who had written the scenes of my life. I wondered why I had so many tragedies, why so much pain, and ongoing suffering. For what purpose? Surely all my choices didn't bring this level of torment! Deep inside me, a voice stirred. It whispered from the shadows, I was solely responsible. I had once again not listened. I chose a destructive path; one that included self-sabotaging my life.

For years, I had run away and pretended everything was okay, and in essence, that was exactly what I was doing again. I never stayed and faced my fears. Instead, I covered up all my problems and escaped the reality that was presented to me.

My final trip away to Townsville was when I decided it was time to fight again. This time I had two battles to win, one for my health and the other for my relationship. I had been defeated before, but I had more knowledge now. I was stronger, more resilient, and more was at stake. This time, to win, I would have to confront the dark parts of myself, and work towards completely banishing them with reason and self-forgiveness. I knew if I would willingly face my demons, I had the possibility of overcoming their persistent hold over me. By doing this, I hoped that I could restore all that had been stolen from me.

None of it came easily or quickly. It required a lot of time and dedication. Over twelve months, I uncovered and overcame my insecurities, and I tried to rebuild a lost and forgotten world. I vowed to stand in the HCV treatment ring again, this time until the end. No matter how hard I got punched or beaten, I would stand firm in my conviction. I would also try and reignite my relationship. I was once blinded and infatuated with the lure of power and success, but now, the lenses in my new glasses forced me to see the real picture. I sensed the potential my marriage had, and in my mind I relived the gift we shared all those months ago. The gift we both threw away, after our defeat.

The first step was to take full responsibility for my past actions. I accepted these historical events as part of my existence. I chose not to live in my unstable house of cards anymore. I would face the storm of my emotions before my whole dwelling tumbled down around me. I could not afford to lose this battle. It would be won, and it would be a victory for all to see.

Chapter 85

Preparing for battle
"The game of life is not so much in holding a good hand as playing a poor hand well."
- H.T. Leslie

My first objective in the battle plan was to fight for another shot at treatment. Time had armed me with knowledge, the latest research, and the skill of my previous journey. I now knew I was what they called a slow responder, and I required eighteen months of treatment. I was so close last time. If only I knew what I knew now, back then......

I knew this new journey would be arduous, but I was mentally prepared to do whatever it took. My persistence paid off and I was offered a place with my well known ally, my previous, friendly gastroenterologist.

I believe when we face challenges in life that are far beyond our own power, it is an opportunity to build on our faith as well as our inner strength and courage. I couldn't control the cards I was dealt. What I did control was my attitude. I learnt to master change rather than allowing it to master me. I came to understand that my attitude affected my life both positively and negatively.

I learnt that my attitude was more important than anything. It was a lot more important than appearances, money, knowledge, or skill. Attitudes can break people. They can destroy families just as my attitude and misguided beliefs did. A remarkable choice is presented to us each day. Which attitude will we embrace? Will it be one of compassion and forgiveness, or one of criticism or blame? I no longer took on the latter because I witnessed first-hand the destruction they could cause. I realised I was the only one in control of my attitude. No one else had that authority. I came to understand just what a difference a positive attitude could make. Adopting a positive attitude changed every aspect of my life.

I started to make preparations for the next round of treatment. I quit my job and secured an executive position with a company that assisted drug addicts by providing support, welfare, education, health care and counselling. Although I knew this position included state-wide duties, the company offered more support and understanding than the previous one. It was a strategic move, and one I was content and satisfied with. I allowed myself three months to establish myself within the organization, before I commenced treatment. I was glad I had done that, I really did need that settling-in period as the workplace was volatile, turbulent and unpredictable, but great.

> *"It is clearly not the journey for everyone. People succeed in as many ways as there are people. Some can be completely fulfilled with destinations that are much closer to home and more comfortable. But if you long to keep going, then I hope you are able to follow my lead to the places I have gone. To be within a whisper of your own personal perfection. To places that are sweeter because you worked so hard to arrive there. To places at the very edge of your dreams."*
>
> *- Michael Johnson*

Chapter 86

An empty harbour
"Every human being has a work to carry on within, duties to perform abroad, influence to exert, which are peculiarly his, and which no conscience but his own can teach."
- William Ellery Channing

Treatment started again in November 2008 and would continue through till April 2009. Eighteen months stood ahead of me, a daunting prospect. It would be a relentless and arduous task for anyone to bear, but I was ready, all my preparation in place. I realised this would be a lonely journey, radically different from my last session. My marriage was in ruins. We were a union in name only. Our love and ongoing friendship helped us to create an illusion to the outside world. However, I knew in my heart I would sail my ship alone this time. There would be no support for me, as John was mentally removed from the situation, caught up in his own career.

So, my ship set sail, much better equipped and well-organized this time, ready for the extensive eighteen-month voyage. Its cargo complete with prescribed amounts of harmful chemicals, as well as supporting naturopathic aids. I plotted a solitary course on the vast ocean where I knew loneliness would reside and surround me.
I perceived what solitude was, but not how far it would extend in my life. As I travelled the highway of treatment, I walked amongst bustling streets crammed with people, but a crowd does not offer company. I came to realise we were just primates who all moved in the same jungle, and our communication processes were sometimes just undecipherable sounds that no one cared to try and understand. Loneliness is hard to bear when you are a social creature, and I missed the company and affection that was once mine a long time ago.

Every morning my ritual began with tablets, followed by a long drive to work, then the pretence of wellness and the ongoing attempt to not show any sign of illness. My façade never wavered. I kept my plight to myself. I learnt to live inside myself, in a safe place, where I could renew my own springs of life-giving water by reading the

Bible and praying.

My husband created and lived a new life for himself. He was physically present, but no longer mentally by my side. He offered minimal assistance and support. His new career challenged him, demanded long hours, which prevented him from engaging with me on any level. His desire to rebuild a life with me faltered as every day passed, and I was too ill to try.

We were both disastrous actors who were scripted to play a part from a Shakespearean tragedy. The scenes portrayed very delicate deep emotions, but neither of us was capable of understanding our situation or how to change the circumstances to improve our lives. Our ships had individually left the harbour, yet bonds of time, twenty-four years of history, still tightly anchored us together in the same port. At the end of each day, both of us returned to the same marina, a haven to shelter together from the outside storms.

"Nothing causes a more decisive defeat than a negative attitude. When you are confronted with a challenge and imagine it is absolutely impossible to overcome you have already lost the battle. This happens when you gauge your troubles against your capabilities. Focus on your victory and God's ability to get you there. You have been given the courage you need for the challenge ahead, now use it."

Marcus Aurelius

Chapter 87

Destructive forces at work

"Constant kindness can accomplish much. As the sun makes ice melt, kindness causes misunderstanding, mistrust and hostility to evaporate."
Kahlil Gibran

Six months into my treatment program, the ground realigned itself with earth shattering force. It not only moved, it pounded both our lives from all sides. I was temporarily working in Cairns when I received a message that my sister-in-law had been taken to hospital with a suspected liver problem. She was, at that time, just having tests. No thorough diagnosis had been given, so I maintained my schedule and returned home the following day.
Upon my homecoming, I contacted my brother-in-law for an update.

He was genuinely distressed and troubled by her now pronounced condition. A harsh reality had struck him fully in the face. His words barely escaped his lips before his weeping began. She had been diagnosed with liver cancer, and her mortality advanced very quickly. So quickly, in fact, that treatment was not an option. She had been placed in a clinical hospital room, waiting only for death to take her. The words were unexpected, and they pierced me heart. I had only seen her a few weeks ago, and she looked happy and healthy. I would never have guessed she was terminally ill. I had no indication at all.

I drove straight to the hospital with my unpacked bags still in the car. I hadn't eaten anything all morning, and my empty stomach screamed for attention. Fatigue overwhelmed me, as it had been a crazy, hectic few days in Cairns. We had launched a new program and visited numerous local services, and my body ached all over, the toll of my treatment regime. I couldn't focus on my problems. I needed to see my sister-in-law. I quickly walked down the well-lit hall and stopped at the nurses' station to inquire which room she was in.

As I neared the door to her room, I was struck by a smell, a sickly sweet, overpowering odour, which permeated the air all around me. It assaulted my lungs and brought the nausea I had fought all day to the surface. When I looked in, I noticed she was sitting on her designated cot, dressed in street clothing. The white, heavily starched bed linen rustled beneath her fragile weight as she twisted to greet me. Her single room was clean and sterile. A window offered a view of a tiny well-manicured garden, which was unseen from where her bed was positioned. Stark white walls devoid of any emotion surrounded her.

I knew I had to change her room, modify it, make it homier, more alive and inviting. Its current bareness depressed me, and I didn't have to spend the rest of my time on earth in it. I recalled I had large, laminated pictures of Norfolk Island, Vanuatu and Hawaii, as well as other beautiful landscapes at home, somewhere. I would find them and bring them in and strategically place them around her. I would also buy some flowering plants to create a more pleasant environment.

Her husband affectionately stroked her arm, whilst they shared a special moment. Her laughter filled the air and made me smile. I stood at the end of the bed and mentally captured every picture. My mind catalogued the scene. The comparison between the once vibrant beautiful woman I knew and the one I saw now was vastly different. She wore a disease-ravaged body, with yellow skin and piercing eyes that glowed. Liquid cysts rose and fell with her every breath, but she still managed to smile at me all the same.

I kissed her and asked how she was going. We talked and I tried to process the landscape before me. The outlook was not optimistic and both of us knew the end was near. I spent the rest of her conscious time pretending to be a hospital jester. I wanted laughter and fun to surround her. I helped her recall wonderful and happy moments in her life, and brought some cheerfulness into this depressing situation.

I visited her every day until her death, eight days later. I decorated her room with flowers, plants and pictures of places she had been, and dreamed of going. We talked about travelling, building dreams, both knowing they would never come to fruition. I continued this until her mind surrendered to the void between life and death, a place where speech to the living was no longer heard. It was a place where her body was unyielding and trapped in an internal war. Caught in a fight she would inevitably lose.

I watched her suffer daily, as she battled to live. I saw a reflection of my own potential death. If I did not clear this virus this time, what would be my options? Would I end up like her, dying in pain, in an isolated, unhomely, sterile room? This was liver cancer. A cancer that threatened me. I watched it as it slowly stole a life right in front of me. I already had cirrhosis. Liver cancer was the next progression. Would this happen to me if I didn't clear this virus? Would I die like this? This thought horrified me. It literally freaked me out!

Even though the cavern between us deepened with every breath she laboriously took, I maintained my vigilance. My one-sided conversations were filled with words of love and the gift of God's grace. The nurses encouraged me to continue to talk to her, informing me that the hearing sense is the last sense to go. This restored my confidence in my belief that she could understand what I said.

During this time, I struggled internally with my own fears. However, it also made me realise just how much I had to live for, and just how much I actually wanted to live.

My life had changed. I had changed. There was still so much I wanted to do, and I didn't want it taken from me by this disease or a cancer that crept silently up on me to steal everything I had ever wanted. I knew my mind was strong and getting stronger by the day. I would use it to visualise my liver as it got healthier, and the virus as it shrivelled up and died within me.

> **"Look within, for within is the wellspring of virtue, which will not cease flowing, if you cease not from digging."**
>
> *Unknown*

Chapter 88

Winds blow from every side
"We are God's workmanship, created to do good works which has been prepared in advance."
Ephesians 2:10

Just before my sister-in-law's diagnosis, my brother-in-law was also diagnosed with aggressive prostate cancer. I had tried to assist him by attending the specialist appointment with him so that he could make an informed decision. My health background enabled me to aid and offer support to him in comprehending the information provided. After deliberating over all the options, he chose to have surgery, and this was pre-scheduled. Unfortunately, his surgery date fell on the same date as his sister's entry into hospital.

I felt torn between the two siblings. I knew it was impossible to support both of them simultaneously, so I decided to sit beside the one I knew for sure was terminal. She also lived in the same city as me, and I would maintain vigilance by phone for the other one. I was lucky my working conditions were flexible enough to enable me to work from the hospital room. I tried to spend every spare moment with her that I could.

During this traumatic time, John, my tragically lost friend and lover, returned mentally and physically to our marriage. He chose to fully reengage in our life, but this was short lived. Life without your best friend is like living on a deserted island. Our short re-engagement enabled us to multiply the good in our lives, and divide up the unpleasantness. We fleetingly shared the pain and the sorrow of the moment, but unfortunately, it didn't last.

Two siblings fought simultaneously together, both faced fatal illnesses. One would go on for the next eighteen months, and battle fearlessly for his life, plagued by complications from his surgery. He required more hospital stays, more surgery, rehabilitation and counselling to regain his life. The other would lose her life.

John was unable to cope with the plight of his two siblings as well as a wife fighting the battle for her life and undergoing a lengthy treatment regime. All of this forced John to wander alone into another alternative dimension, like something out of The Talisman by Stephen King, a story of a boy who remained the same, but had the opportunity to run away into a parallel universe. John sought happiness and joy to replace the doom and gloom of the real world. Unknown to me at the time, John started to live a dual existence; one where he was the family man, and the other where he was the player on the internet chat rooms, where he could pretend to be something unreal, a fictional character that in reality he was not.

"A moment's insight is sometimes worth a life's experience."

- Oliver Wendell Holmes

Chapter 89

Tragedy strikes
"Great opportunities to help others seldom come, but small ones surround us every day."
- Sally Koch

The final hours approached. Preparations had been made, family members were called, and still she grasped life with all her strength. She held on. She battled and seized every moment. Every breath was laboured as her heart and lungs struggled to feed a dying body. The doctors and nurse were impressed by her strength, but I wondered why she would wage such a war. I was told she was most likely waiting for someone. Besides her husband, only my children had engaged with her during this, her final crusade.

Her mother and sister lived one and a half hours away on the Gold Coast, and unfortunately, both chose to stay by the brother's side, even though they were aware she was terminally ill. Like a medic on a battlefield conducting triage, the choice was where to spend one's time. Who do you devote time and energy to? The doomed or the injured? In this case, both appeared doomed. John's brother was in intensive care with the real possibility of dying any day as well. He was divorced and had no partner. John's sister was married, and her partner was beside her. How does a mother choose between two dying children? I hoped I would never have to make such a decision.

Like many families, the years, and a series of incidents, had caused rifts in their cohesion as a family unit. Miscommunications, unresolved issues which stemmed from childhood and adolescence choices and behaviours, as well as personality clashes and expectations not met, all those familiar catalysts that occur over the years amongst siblings and parents, were present in this family as well. John had naturally known some reasons for their dysfunctionality, but was not able to fix himself, let alone everyone else.

I, personally, couldn't understand why her mother did not visit. A coherent answer eluded me. What unknown tragedies and afflictions had affected this family, that none would come now, and see this family member? What rifts could cause such reactions and decisions? I only knew of my own devastating childhood and adolescence. John's explanations of his family dysfunctions were never fully explained or uncovered.

Even as I tried to understand and process these things, a fire burned within me, a fury I could not stop. It burnt fiercely, and I found it hard to quench. I knew I needed to douse their flames as it was not the time for inappropriate behaviour on my part.

I was tired from my extended stays and trying to work within the hospital setting. I needed a break. I rang her mother and pleaded with her to come, to be with her daughter. I explained the situation and informed her of what the doctors had rationalized, about why she would not let go, even though she was in immense pain. Relief swept over me, tears filled my eyes, as she finally agreed to come.

I was physically exhausted, unsure how much longer I could maintain this level of effectiveness. My treatment and hospital regime and my lack of sleep and limited nutrition, as well as trying to maintain my management position and complete the last two modules of my Masters, were all taking their toll.

The phone call over, and with reinforcements set to arrive shortly, I started to uncontrollably weep. My sobs echoed down the long empty corridor, breaking the silence. My grief and tension was able to be truly released, freed from its oppression.

I counted down the hours to my liberation. My bedridden companion's continuous laboured breathing provided a constant steady rhythm, as my fingers hit the keyboard of my laptop, and my mind created a new program for work. The smell of her pungent sweat surrounded me, and her infrequent small whimpers and sighs, periodically distracted me. My mobile buzzed in my pocket, notifying me of the family's arrival. I was thankful, grateful, that they had come. I hoped this woman who lay on the bed, dying, could now finally find peace.

However, I was shocked to find only her sister had come. My

mother-in-law failed to appear. This left a dark shadow in a space only a mother's presence could fill. My heart sank. I was confounded and shocked by her absence, her choice a complete mystery to me.

I called her, and again I pleaded for her to come. A mother's plea, from a mother to another mother. I held my mobile to her daughter's ear, with the hope she would at least be able to hear and comprehend her mother's words of endearment as they passed to her dying child. I begged again, and finally she accepted. She said she would arrive that night. I had won a battle. A battle that should never have been fought. It was no victory for me. The triumphant moment was solely for a beautiful, unconscious girl.

The family was fully reunited, bar one; a brother who fought in an ICU for his own life, elsewhere. I left them to make peace. I had said my final goodbye. A glorious, yet sorrowful point in time, and I went home and slept a fit, full sleep, my conflict over. I knew I had done the best I could. I had done everything possible to make her last journey as good as it could be, under the circumstances.

She died, willingly relinquishing her spirit in my husband's presence early the next morning.

"Though this life may be gone in a week or today, you will forever be alive in the hearts of those who love you & will live forever in heaven until we see each other again in the presence of our Holy God".

- Kodee Williams

Chapter 90

Destructive paths destroy lives
"We do not remember days, we remember moments".
- Cesare Pavese

Life moved from hours to days to weeks. We were all temporarily trapped in our sadness. John suffered more than I did, but both our grieving changed us in unimaginable ways. My husband withdrew more and more into himself. He decided to choose a voluntary madness of inebriation and the devious forces it brought with it. Mischievous spirits consumed, enticed and allured him from every angle, and he was weak and led down a very destructive path.

Me, I became more obsessed and addicted to my work. I devoted every waking hour to it, forfeiting everything else. I withdrew from everyone, my friends and family included. I hid my grief within myself, behind a rebuilt wall of my castle. One of my friends never gave up on me. She repeatedly tried to reach out to me, and she often quoted, "Laurie, you know people are lonely because they build walls instead of bridges."

I knew she was right, but I just didn't have the strength to combat my grief as well as try to survive the ride of treatment and work, and to nurture my family and friends. It just wasn't in me right now. So I left the nurturing part out, for now. She was rather philosophical, as she would tell me I couldn't change the direction of the wind, but what I could adjust was my sails to accommodate it. I understood the message she was referring to; my attitude. But I really didn't think I had the energy to sustain any sort of relationship with anyone. I found just living was hard enough for me.

John worked constantly. I hardly saw him or spent any time with him. I made myself too busy to care. After all, I was trying to combat the side effects of a harsh treatment as well as a disease I knew could potentially kill me if I didn't take care of myself. I had just witnessed how fast liver cancer could strike, and kill you. I watched its burning fingers eat away at a life that had much more to offer to this world.

I spent many nights alone, which enabled me to reflect on many things in my life. One of which was this treatment journey and the vast difference between the two bouts. My initial forty-eight week regime was wholly supported by a loving husband, who regularly massaged my aching body, ran aromatherapy baths for me, cooked and made juices for me, stroked my body, and tried to take the pain away. He even covered some of my shifts at work when I was too tired or sick to attend. This bout was a lonely, unsupported and demanding seventy-two week journey. A gruelling battle I alone endured. I attended all my appointments unaccompanied. He didn't seem to care. He was so caught up in his own world, a world I didn't belong in. What a difference five years and an illness can make to a marriage! This rejection from him instigated a complete shut down between us, and I placed work in the void I felt. Work became my safe haven, where I felt accepted, needed and appreciated.

A perpetual cycle was set in motion when I didn't clear the virus the first time. We were both so disappointed and devastated, the strain damaged our relationship and caused a rift to grow between us. Our love was far from gone. It was just lost in the chasm that had formed between us. We needed each other like the desert needs the rain, but neither of us sought the oasis that would have saved us. Both of us ran the same eighteen-month marathon, but we did it as competitors against each other, as two lost souls. We sought the same goal, but our iPods drowned out the reality of how we could do it more efficiently, together.

Towards the end of this long journey, I had started to realise just how estranged we had become. I felt the loss deep in my heart. Pictures of our lives in much happier circumstances flowed easily through my mind. They brought a smile to my lips, but a tear to my eye. They made me question, what had gone wrong? What did I do?

I knew I had pushed him away. And, for the first time, I really looked and saw through his behaviour. I saw the needs of his heart and I realised I had never met any of these needs. My independence, self-reliance, my hardened heart and inflexible nature had caused the first fissures to form in our relationship a long time ago. Treatment had just closed them up, sealing us inside. What did I expect? A person can only take so much rejection. I realised just how I had contributed to this void that lay between us. I just had to figure out what to do about it and how to get back to where we once were.

"Good timber does not grow with ease. The stronger the wind the stronger the trees."

- Williard Marriott

Chapter 91

My bronze crown
"In the end, a person is only known by the impact they have on others."
- Jim Stovall

In October 2009, eleven months after I started my second regime of treatment, I kicked my first goal. I had won a major battle. A bronze crown now lay upon my head. My tests informed me the treatment was working. I had cleared the virus! The virus was undetectable in my blood. I was not yet able to stand on the podium and receive my gold crown, but I was one step closer to this cherished accolade. I could see it, taste it, feel it upon my skin, and I vowed to receive it.

This news lifted my spirits. I was like an eagle that soared above the clouds. It was excellent news, incomparable. However, being genotype 1a1b and a slow responder, I still faced another six months of the bombardment of chemicals. However, nothing would stand in my way of the glory that would be mine. Pegasys bombs could merrily explode within me, for my mental defence had been reinforced and reinstated.

A new optimism inspired my faith, defeated my hopelessness, rid me of my internal despair and it dared me to believe that I may live a normal, long life; one not overshadowed by HCV. Up until this point I was convinced I had no definite certainty in my life, no guarantees or assurances, no dependability. Nothing was constant or solid. Could I possibly still be here in another five, ten years? Did I dare to dream again, make plans for a noteworthy future?

Were all my prayers finally answered? Had God listened to me? It appeared unquestionable, crystal-clear. Could I now start to rebuild my shattered world? My Father would often tell me, "Laurie, God can take the bits and pieces of your un-reached goals, and put them back together again. He takes the shattered fragments of your life and restores them to wholeness."

He also told me God can take the fragments of what I once believed, and make them as new and fresh as the dawning sun. Was that a possibility? Could He restore my health? My relationship? Was that possible? At times, I would ask Dad why he thought this was happening. His answer was simple, "we are all still at school. Gods school. Sometimes the lessons are tough, but we are here on earth to learn and teach others. Graduation only really occurs when we die."

My journey had already taught me so much about life, and about myself. How much more was there? I knew I had not used the previous lessons I had learnt wisely. I had gone back to a lot of my old familiar behaviours, backsliding in to the pit and sabotaging all the relationships around me. I pushed people away and reconstructed my castle walls. I also played with the skills of the chameleon. Maybe it was time to be honest and allow people to see the real me. Maybe, just maybe, it was time to become the real Laurie, the person I knew lived within me.

> *"The important thing is not to stop questioning. Curiosity has its own reason for existing. One cannot help but be in awe when he contemplates the mysteries of eternity, of life, of the marvellous structure of reality."*
>
> *- Albert Einstein*

Chapter 92

A will to live

"Don't be afraid that your life will end, be afraid that it will never begin."
- *anonymous*

My life changing news arrived a week before my father had a serious heart attack. I rushed to his side to assist as he was taken to a remote hospital, and then airlifted to Prince Charles Hospital for triple bypass surgery.

John and I aptly named 2009 "the year of the hospital." The year had started with his sister's death, and then his brother's numerous bouts of surgery, which at times required lengthy stays in hospital, and now, my dad. Three events. One ended in tragedy and two battled on.

My father fought arduously for his life. His recovery was long and problematic. The surgery a success, but his body and mind struggled under the torrent of medications and the confinement that hospital entails. His belief that pharmaceutical drugs were poison made it hard for the medical staff to positively address all his needs. His extended stay also induced a depressed state in him.

I would sit everyday with the man I had come to adore, and attempt to revitalize and renew his failing spirits. Many a night we would discuss our treatment, our health and our future plans. We daydreamed of spending time in Cairns together, taking holidays and building many more memories. I placed inspirational posters around him, surrounding him with messages of love and hope. I also plastered his room with vibrant pictures of Cairns and a place called Paranella Park, in the hope of creating a liveable dream within him. Paranella Park was a place I had previously visited, and I promised to take him there when he was well enough to travel. I watched as he slowly created a mental picture of this, and a smile rose to his lips for the first time in nearly a month.

His low point came one night when I was with him. He had simply had enough of the tubes, the medications and the loss of dignity. The time in hospital, for him, now unbearable. He could see no light at the end of the tunnel. His future had become a vision that was blurry in the distance. I sat on the cold, tiled floor beside him. I held his hand and spoke of a time many months ago, when I was so desperate, so disgusted in myself that I was ready to finish my life.

We shared a moment and we cried together. We both knew just how close each of us had truly come to giving up. As I drove away from the hospital towards home, I realised just how vulnerable we all are, and just how precious life actually is.

Not long after this, he was released from hospital. He had triumphed over his adversity. His skirmish with the initial throes of death was finally over. However, he would engage in a battle to survive, struggling with an enemy for another eight months.

Six months later, as I was nearing the end of my treatment, we went to Cairns for a holiday, and we did visit Paranella Park.

"Imagination is more important than knowledge. Imagination is what we could be."

- Albert Einstein

Chapter 93

Footprints in the sand
*Cherish things while you still have them, before they're gone,
and you realize how precious they really are.*
- *Author unknown*

Days fell into a steady rhythm. A consistent pattern emerged around me. Treatment a ceaseless hum constantly in the background of every situation, nausea a continual reminder of the phase I was in. I had now lost eighteen kilograms. My hormones played havoc with my moods and bodily functions. I found it hard to function outside of work. I was more aggressive and I had absolutely no social life.

My energy levels were so low, I needed to rest frequently. I had become quite breathless, and my body, especially my hips, ached constantly with a deep penetrating throb which hindered my movements. My beloved exercise regime had become non-existent. Sleep persistently eluded me, yet I was so tired, both physically and mentally weary. Pain burned deep within my muscles. Its fingers persistently stabbed me. Acid blazed up the long tube of my oesophagus, bringing a smouldering agony. It prevented me from lying down for any length of time. Most nights, in the darkest hours, I would get up and work, or go for a walk, eager for some form of relief. Hours later, totally exhausted and still in pain, I would fall back into bed and try to gain some strength to face the challenges of the new day.

My life became a ritual of going to work and trying to survive the day. Some days were harder than others. I chose to "fly under the radar" so to speak, so nobody would notice how ill I was. Then, I would come home to an empty house, an empty bed and I would watch a little mind-numbing television. Each morning I would prepare my disguise. The drive to work offered me just enough time to cover my decaying essence with a stoic, manageable smile.

John and I were not always estranged. At times, when our rosters aligned, we would share unique, loving moments. However, our relationship was not as intimate. It was strangely guarded. I felt John had pulled away and was caught, trapped in a cave with no easily found exit. I felt that he held himself back from me, but I was too sick to comprehend what was happening right in front of me, as my focus was on getting through treatment.

We were once passionately together. Now, we were cohabitants that enjoyed a deep, mutual friendship. What I really missed was the companionship. My heart knew where it belonged It didn't understand the restriction of treatment. It just knew it was painfully chained up, confined. To lose someone you love alters your life forever. No one can fill their place in your heart. Their particular energy is unique, irreplaceable, and it leaves a gap that never closes. Some people are transients in life; they touch us then quickly move on. Others stay and leave footprints in the sands of your soul, which change us forever. John had left a mark on me; one I would never be able to erase. A mark I didn't want to erase. When I said my vows to him in 1988, I meant them.

I don't believe that love ever dies a natural death. It dies simply because it is not nurtured or replenished. It dies, slowly affected by betrayals, blindness, significant illnesses, wounds that penetrate deeply and the weariness of life. I knew we were close to losing everything. I felt it deep within me. However, I believed and stood firm to the convictions that we could have a great future together. Now that I knew I had a future, without HCV, I was not going to live it without the man who had fought for our relationship so courageously just a few years before.

I had previously given up on everything in life, but, thankfully people didn't give up on me. Their prayers and support from a distance assisted me continually. I was not prepared to throw the towel into the arena, conceding my marriage was over, because I knew it wasn't, especially now when we were so near to the summit.

We had travelled so far, been through so much. We had just been at different universities learning individualised lessons, and meeting and working with different people. My teachers were more from a counselling background who supported, guided and nurtured my self-development, whereas his were from the school of hard knocks, promoting and encouraging poor choices. I was taught to positively reach the summit, and not to give up as the summit was now well within my reach, and I needed to stand strong and fight for the life I wanted.

Whilst I was at my university, I attended in-depth painting lessons. I know that sounds funny, but, I did. To paint, you need to really learn to see more clearly. Seeing is more than just looking at something. It is discerning the deeper essence of what's presented before you, assessing every part individually and comprehending beyond what's obviously seen. People are the same; their deeper meaning needs to be uncovered. They need to be explored, peeled back layer by layer and offered acceptance. People are more than the colours and textures they present on the surface. Inside them exists unique qualities, hidden talents and wonderful histories. I learnt to see John in this manner. I saw the hurts, the pain, the rejection and the barriers he had constructed to protect himself. I saw his vulnerabilities, and this made me love him more. I learnt to see past what was being presented to me on the surface and started to explore the layers underneath. I also started to use this technique to look deep within myself.

In effect, I sincerely saw my whole life from another perspective, and the picture was not what I had expected. I knew I had embraced the darker shadows in my life, and had carried a heavy burden. What I didn't recognise was just how self-destructive I had been. During the long months of treatment, especially the last six months, I learnt, with the help of a few mentors, to offload my burdens, and replace them with positive affirmations and more constructive behaviours, and my life began to hold real meaning.

> *"Destiny is not a matter of chance, it is a matter of choice; it is not a thing to be waited for, it is a thing to be achieved. A journey of a thousand miles begins with a single step."*
>
> *Author unknown*

Chapter 94

A fearful moment
It isn't what you have in your pocket that makes you thankful, but what you have in your heart.
- Unknown

For the last forty-eight weeks, and the forty-four weeks before it, John had safely administered my interferon injection. However, he received a needle stick injury one night, as he was placing the needle into the disposal bin, which was very full. It appeared that a needle had turned upside down, and, due to the fullness, had protruded slightly from the top. This is what stabbed John in the thumb, causing a deep puncture wound, which immediately started bleeding.

We were both stunned. I immediately told him to make it bleed, squeezing it repeatedly, whilst holding it under cold water, to allow the blood to flow freely. My mind processed the odds of exposure and the risk to him from infection. We didn't know how long the needle had been there. I had been virus free for a couple of months so, his risks were small, but there was still a risk. I didn't really want to think about it.

I silently questioned just how long the needle would have been in there. Was it fresh? I knew the virus weakened and died within 72 hours, it also doesn't like sunlight, preferring a dark, humid environment. Even though I weighed all these facts up, I was still anxious that I may have infected him. The fact I was no longer infected was a distinctive plus, but there was still an element of doubt in my mind.

We bandaged up the wound, and I rang my work colleague, a male counsellor who could talk to John about his risk factors. I could not suppress the feelings of hopelessness and dread, and I allowed them to flow freely through me. Anxious, uneasy tears comforted me at night, and fear and worry troubled me during the day, whilst I waited for the results to come in. I would not totally succumb to them this time. They could have their moment, but that would be all I would allow.

Laurie Smyth

John's outside wound healed, but his heart hardened, as he waited for his pending test results. We certainly didn't need any more mayhem or chaos in our lives right now. I didn't think I could handle any more turmoil. I just wanted peace, tranquillity and space to restore order in all this disorder.

I read somewhere that a person can live forty days without food, but only three days without water. However, if we have no hope, we can't live at all, not one second. I couldn't believe that this journey was all for nothing, that I would lose everything now. I had lived my whole life full of fear. Fear of rejection, not being worthy, not smart enough, and that was all changing. The way I felt about myself was different. The way I felt about everything in my life was different. I appreciated things, people, situations - including this journey I was on now.

Looking back, I can see that for most of my adult life, I was never one hundred percent present in any relationship. I always held a part of me back, the part I feared would get broken, my heart. Five years ago, that started to change. I started to let my guard down, and I witnessed something magical. Something I had never experienced before, real love. And, I fell in love.

The pit that threatened me yet again was deep and dark, but I now had a different but definite foothold; a reliable aid to help me claw my way to the top. The surface's bright light illuminated my path. I was determined to win. I propelled myself upwards. Misfortunes, disappointments and setbacks would not prevent me this time from taking and having the life I knew was possible. I was really ready to fight for my life. I saw the potential in it. The things I had once dreamed of were tangible now, and I would not be beaten by a needle stick injury and the guilt that surrounded it.

I don't believe circumstances happen by chance. Every little occurrence holds a deeper meaning. Our eyes are sometimes clouded by our perceptions. This can prevent us from seeing things clearly, but if we seek further and expand our perspective, maybe even look outside the box, so to speak, eventually, all is revealed. I didn't understand what was happening in my life, but I believed it would be revealed to me when I was ready and could understand and deal with it.

John's first HCV test was negative, as were his second and third tests. I was extremely relieved. John didn't say too much, although I knew he was also relieved. I couldn't dwell on his behaviour, as I had to focus on mine, and finish the marathon I was on.

I realised all I really had was today. Right now, this very moment was really all I could control. It was unproductive and a waste of time to dwell on what happened yesterday, or in the past, or even what was coming in the future. I had no control over any of it, the only thing I could control was my attitude and how I made people feel.

My life was like a building project. The block of units I designed didn't go up over night, but by using due diligence, they were created, and I knew my efforts today would help create tomorrow's results.

And I would wait for John to see the changes in me, and to hopefully reengage in our relationship.

> *Each new day is a new beginning-*
> *to learn more about ourselves*
> *to care more about others,*
> *to laugh more than we did,*
> *to accomplish more than we thought we could,*
> *and be more than we were before.*
>
> *-Author Unknown*

Chapter 95

Flowers in full bloom

> *The last, if not the greatest, of the human freedoms:*
> *to choose their own attitude in any given circumstance.*
> **- Bruno Bettelheim**

April had arrived, I entered the arena for the final victory lap, my last self-administered injection, and my last five tablets were taken. I had made it. The battle completed, eighteen long months. I looked back at it with pride. It was the hardest, toughest experience I had ever faced, and it was now conquered, lying behind me. I felt unshackled, released from my bondage. Joy completely surrounded me. I was ecstatic the fight was finally over, euphoria flooded through me. I could live again!

I had adhered to the highest dose of ribavirn all the way through, not changing and not missing a single day. This was something that differentiated this treatment from the last bout. Even though this was a hard task, the science had proven that higher doses of Ribavin enhanced clearance rates, and I wanted to be set free. I had made my mind up to continue on the highest dose, regardless of any symptoms. I was lucky that my blood stabilized at week forty-eight, which enabled me to physically continue on this harsh regime. I was anaemic, tired and rundown, but none of that mattered now. I chose to continue because I knew the benefits far outweighed the costs.

The arduous trek over, I adopted an attitude of pure joy, savouring every experience. Exhilaration radiated out of me with the force of an atomic bomb, and it surrounded everyone and everything I came in contact with.

Once I re-found laughter, I knew I could survive any painful situation that may come my way in the future, and with humour, I learnt I could soften some of the catastrophic strikes that life delivered. Life is about change. We can't stop it, just as we can't stop the earth from spinning, but what we can change is how we deal with the situation and how we treat others. For me, a healthy attitude, as well as the ability to forgive and not hold onto things is how I brought joy and contentment back into my life. I have heard a statement that many people die at twenty-five, but are not buried till they are seventy. I didn't want to live my life like that. Before this journey, I believe that could possibly have been me.

I can honestly say, I am glad I went through it. I am grateful for my life, I am grateful for the people that surround me, I am grateful that I am loved, and I am grateful that I have been given a second chance, and I am so grateful that I am not the same person I was five years ago.

Thankyou God

Chapter 96

The crown is finally mine to keep
"In this world, there is no clarity. There is only love and action."
- Mother Teresa

In October, I had cleared the virus. It was now late April, and I was due for the first of three PCR tests. I was encouraged by the negative results of six months ago, but I wondered if it would be sustainable. The wait for these results was really tough. I questioned whether or not I would fail again. On the surface, I was optimistic, but underneath lay my true fear. The depths of it rose in waves. What would happen to me and my relationship, if I didn't clear the virus? We were already on the brink of a break up, passion between us long gone, replaced by indifference, apathy and selfishness. Where would my life take me if I didn't clear? I dare not dream of a life worth living, not yet.

I couldn't wait any longer, so I went to see my Egyptian GP to get the result. My husband, no longer interested in my plight, left me to seek the results alone. His coldness and unresponsiveness struck a blow to my heart, wounding it deeply.

The waiting room was, as always, overcrowded and busy, filled with anxious people seeking solace in trashy magazines and the gossip they held. My nervousness prevented me from focusing on anything but the door that hid my results. As I sat amongst the noise and confusion, I promised myself to move forward no matter what the conclusion today. My determination was to stand steadfast, not succumbing to the afflictions and despair of the past. I would completely strip myself of my old habits, behaviours, attitudes and beliefs, and replace them with the new person I had become. Today would symbolize a brand new beginning. Either way, I would start again, despite what was said today.

The door opened and there he stood, his Egyptian welcoming gaze fell on my anxious, upturned face. His smile broadened and lit up his entire face. His hands at once ushered me into his congested office. I sat and faced him. My eyes searched the computer screen as they sought my results.

He knew exactly why I was there, and he wasted no time providing me with my answer. He turned, his face animated, beaming. He congratulated me. Telling me I had finally done it. I jumped up, unable to contain my excitement, embracing him and thanking him. What a joyous moment this was! My heart pounded like a galloping race horse. Elation filled me. I felt like dancing. Pure pleasure emanated from him as he accompanied me to the door, steering me into the waiting room. I glowed as I walked to the counter, and he visually followed, smiling.

I had never felt so happy. I didn't know who to share the news with, so I just started ringing everyone who knew.
That day changed the structures of my whole internal world. Creeping rose bushes brought forth budding beautiful flowers and made their home around my life. The carefree life I had lived so long ago in Madang resurfaced. The same feelings I experienced up there, all those years ago, rose up within me. I saw my future open up with every new bloom. I felt real happiness and joy, and I laughed more than I ever had before.

I would not allow this to be stolen from me again. Not now, not ever.

I made a declaration that I would not look back, guaranteeing only to focus on a bright, positive future. My oath: to do whatever it took to rebuild my life. This would start with my relationship, an intricate undertaking, but not hopeless or unattainable, and worth risking all for. It was time for me to stop acting and to step into the spot light. I was ready to really audition for the role of my life. I would never again be that wounded lioness, as I would become a strong and capable, caring woman.

I decided who I wanted to be in this new life. I had made a choice to be happy and optimistic. My hope was a fire I chose to stoke daily. I learnt that I could not access joy or happiness in tangible things; I had to access it from inside myself. I had previously surrounded myself with stuff that would never make me happy, and I slowly started to remove them, learning to draw on my own internal strengths.

More meaningful interactions with my husband, and others, resulted from this decision, and I stored these positive small milestones on my internal mantel piece. They were like magnets which intensified my efforts to succeed. I had never felt more happy or content in my whole life. I held a constructive, optimistic future in the palm of my hand, and I planned to ride this wave all the way to the beach, again and again, and I would never fall off my surf board again.

My second and third test also came back stating I had been given a second chance. I was no longer emancipated, held to ransom by a disease. I was free, released from my self-imposed imprisonment. Life opened up before me. I stood on a new rock face. I stared at an expanse of water stretched out as far as my eye could see. I could see the rippling, swelling waves that demanded changes. The world was more vivid, more colourful, now the sky had lightened. Nothing was impossible now. The isolated ledge I once stood upon was still a sheer drop, but the dive was now achievable. Diving from this position was no longer impossible. I saw all potential and the promises that lay beneath. The life which I now embraced carried hope, unbound expectations, enlightenment and prospects.

However, in the distance, the darkest clouds loomed ominously, its destructive forces would soon strike, threatening to destroy everything I had achieved, but I would hold steadfast to a promise.

A promise from God.

The best was yet to come.

"Forgiveness is the most powerful thing you can do for yourself. If you can't learn to forgive, you can forget about achieving true success in your life"

- Dr. Dyer

End note

This is the end of this part of my personal expedition. Your journey is also unique and worthy. ***Don't ever forget that.***

If I could impart some wisdom to you, it would be to not give up hope. Never, never give it up! It is what kept me sane and provided strength when I was too weary to ride out the torrential storms that life dealt me.

Never be afraid to sail your own ship, even when the rain blinds you. People surrounding you will always have an opinion. Listen, but do what you need to do.

Fear grows in dark places, so turn on all of your lights. Ask for help, seek a higher power and share with others. Choose to live. Please don't let fear rule your life, fear can rob you of everything!

All your personal experiences provide you with courage and strength. Stop and look fear in the face. Conquer it. It will give up more than it steals from you.

Remember also, what is engraved on your headstone will not be what you are remembered for. What you weave into the fabric of others is what truly matters. Lastly, believe in yourself. You can get to the summit one small step at a time, just don't give in. When you get there, express yourself, yell, scream at whoever deserves it. I couldn't have done this journey without God. You may be different. I needed strength and wisdom to guide me, especially when I was out of control. I believe He showed me the way, and I am so grateful to have Him in my life. I battled with my faith for years, but I have come to realise that it was really all I had.

Remember, you don't have to do this journey alone. Others are here to help you.

God Bless you in your life, and I hope you enjoyed my ride. Thanks for sharing it with me.

MY WISH FOR YOU...

Where there is pain, I wish you peace and mercy. Where there is self-doubting, I wish you a renewed confidence in your ability to work through it. Where there is tiredness, or exhaustion, I wish you understanding, patience, and renewed strength. Where there is fear, I wish you love, and courage.

Visit us on our website
www.hepcandme.com.au

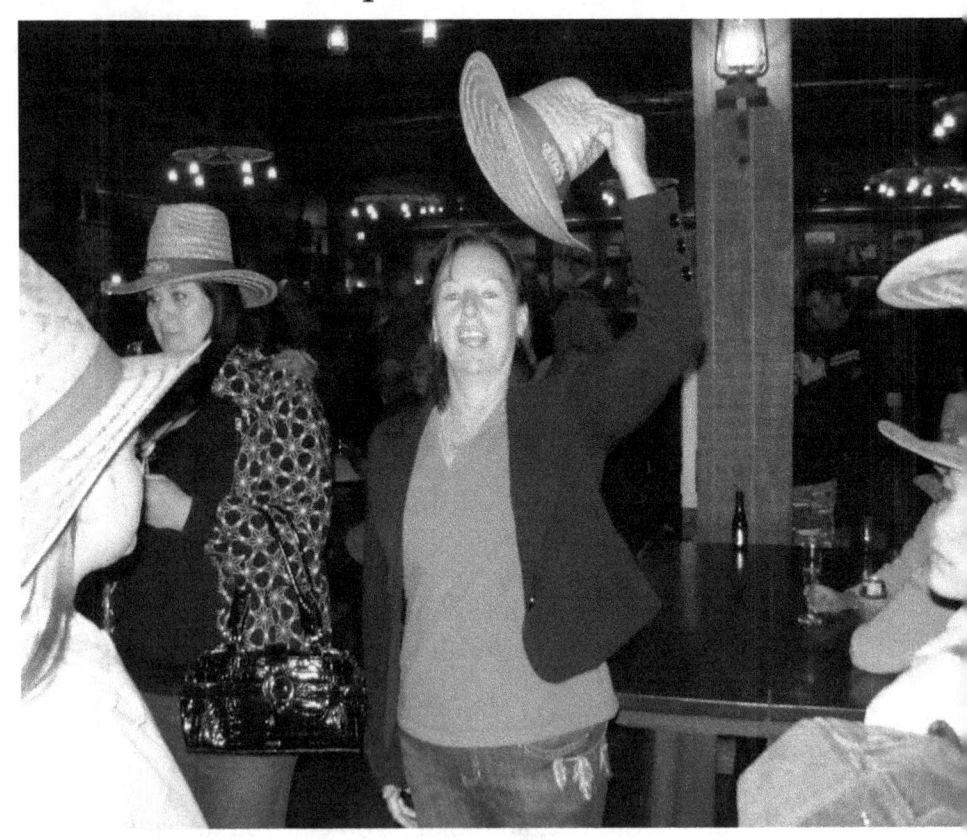

www.ingramcontent.com/pod-product-compliance
Lightning Source LLC
Chambersburg PA
CBHW071708160426
43195CB00012B/1618